A-Z Notes in Radiological Practice and Reporting

Series Editors
Carlo Nicola De Cecco
Andrea Laghi

Giulia Zamboni
Sofia Gourtsoyianni

MDCT and MRI of the Liver, Bile Ducts and Pancreas

Springer

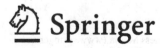

Giulia Zamboni
UOC Radiologia BR
Azienda Ospedaliera
Universitaria Integrata Verona
Verona
Italy

Sofia Gourtsoyianni, MD, PhD
Imaging 2, Level 1
Lambeth Wing
St Thomas' Hospital
London
UK

ISBN 978-88-470-5719-7 ISBN 978-88-470-5720-3 (eBook)
DOI 10.1007/978-88-470-5720-3
Springer Milan Heidelberg New York Dordrecht London

Library of Congress Control Number: 2014955365

Printed on acid-free paper

Springer is part of Springer Science+Business Media (www.springer.com)

Foreword to this Series

A-Z *Notes in Radiological Practice and Reporting* is a new series of practical guides dedicated to residents and general radiologists. The series was born thanks to the original idea to bring to the public attention a series of notes collected by doctors and fellows during their clinical activity and attendance at international academic institutions. Those brief notes were critically reviewed, sometimes integrated, cleaned up, and organized in the form of an A-Z glossary to be usable by a third reader.

The ease and speed of consultation and the agility in reading were behind the construction of this series and were the reasons why the booklets are organized alphabetically, primarily according to disease or condition. The number of illustrations has been deliberately reduced and focused only on those ones relevant to the specific entry.

Residents and general radiologists will find in these booklets numerous quick answers to frequent questions occurring during radiological practice, which will be useful in daily activity for planning exams and radiological reporting.

Each single entry typically includes a short description of pathological and clinical characteristics, guidance on selection of the most appropriate imaging technique, a schematic review of potential diagnostic clues, and useful tips and tricks.

The series will include the most relevant topics in radiology, starting with cardiac imaging and continuing with the gastrointestinal tract, liver, pancreas and bile ducts, and genitourinary apparatus during the first 2 years. More arguments will be covered in the next issues.

The Editors put a lot of their efforts in selecting the most appropriate colleagues willing to exchange with readers their own experiences in their respective fields. The result is a combination of experienced professors, enthusiastic researchers, and young talented radiologists working together within a single framework project with the primary aim of making their knowledge available for residents and general practitioners.
We really do hope that this series can meet the satisfaction of the readers and can help them in their daily radiological practice.

Latina, Italy Carlo Nicola De Cecco
Andrea Laghi

Contents

A

Acute Pancreatitis

Acute pancreatitis is an acute inflammation of the pancreas with variable involvement of other regional tissues or remote organ systems. Mild acute pancreatitis is associated with minimal organ dysfunction, while severe acute pancreatitis is associated with pancreatic necrosis and may lead to organ failure and/or local complications. The most common causes of acute pancreatitis are biliary stones and alcohol abuse, which account for up to 80 % of the cases.

In 2007, the Working Group Classification defined interstitial edematous pancreatitis and necrotising pancreatitis, redefining the terms that should be used to describe the collections present in each phase of the disease.

Interstitial edematous pancreatitis is characterised by a localised or diffuse enlargement of the pancreas, with normal homogeneous enhancement or slightly heterogeneous enhancement due to oedema. There is also mistiness or mild stranding of the peripancreatic fat. The fluid collections present in the early phase are called *acute peripancreatic fluid collections* (*APFC*).

G. Zamboni, S. Gourtsoyianni, *MDCT and MRI of the Liver, Bile Ducts and Pancreas*, A-Z Notes in Radiological Practice and Reporting, DOI 10.1007/978-88-470-5720-3_1,

If these persist longer than 4 weeks, these will become pseudocysts.

In necrotising pancreatitis, areas of pancreatic necrosis appear as hypoattenuating nonenhancing parenchyma. The necrosis can be parenchymal, peripancreatic or both parenchymal and peripancreatic. After 4 weeks, these necrotic collections will develop a wall and become *walled-off necrosis* (*WON or WOPN*).

The revised Atlanta classification has abandoned the terms pancreatic abscess and intrapancreatic pseudocyst, which should not be used anymore.

Adenocarcinoma of the Pancreas

Pancreatic adenocarcinoma (PAC) has a dismal prognosis, with a mortality rate similar to its incidence and an overall 5-year survival rate lower than 5 %. Early diagnosis and resection are the only potential cure, but only a minority (5–30 %) will be diagnosed when still resectable.

CT is the diagnostic procedure of choice in the suspicion of PAC and is a reliable technique for its diagnosis and staging. Ductal adenocarcinoma typically appears as an ill-defined mass, surrounded by extensive desmoplastic reaction. PAC enhances poorly compared to the adjacent normal pancreatic parenchyma, appearing hypodense on arterial phase in most cases (75–90 %: Fig. 1), and may become isodense on delayed imaging.

CT correlates well with surgical findings in predicting unresectability (positive predictive value of 89–100%).

At MRI, PAC appears hypointense to the normal parenchyma on T1-weighted images, with or without fat suppression. On T2-weighted images, the tumour has variable appearance depending on the amount of desmoplastic reaction. After gadolinium administration, PAC usually shows less enhancement compared to the normal parenchyma in the arterial phase. MRI

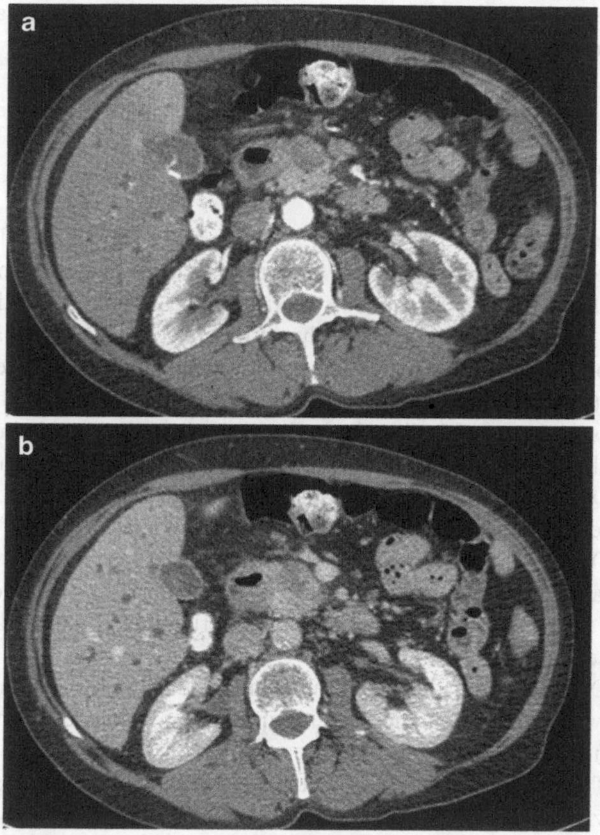

Fig. 1 Axial arterial phase (**a**) and portal-venous phase (**b**) CT images show a solid hypodense lesion in the ventral aspect of the pancreatic head, compatible with pancreatic carcinoma. The fat plane between the lesion and the superior mesenteric vein is preserved. Dilatation of the intrahepatic bile ducts is seen

might visualise up to 79 % of the tumours that appear isodense at CT. Pancreatic carcinoma has a variable appearance on diffusion-weighted images; a high sensitivity and specificity have been reported for DWI in the detection of pancreatic adenocarcinomas.

Adenomyomatosis (Gallbladder)

Adenomyomatosis is a relatively common benign condition, identified in at least 5 % of cholecystectomy specimens. Most often an incidental finding, it frequently coexists with chronic cholecystitis. It is characterised by hypertrophy of the mucosa and muscularis propria and intraluminal cholesterol accumulation. Cholesterol crystals precipitate in the bile trapped in Rokitansky–Aschoff sinuses, intramural diverticula lined by mucosal epithelium. Gallbladder wall thickening and intramural diverticula containing bile with cholesterol crystals, sludge or calculi are the pathologic correlates of the imaging features of adenomyomatosis.

On CT the "rosary sign" has been described, formed by enhancing epithelium within intramural diverticula surrounded by the relatively unenhanced hypertrophied gallbladder muscularis.

On MRI gallbladder wall thickening and T2-w hyperintense, T1-w hypointense, nonenhancing intramural lesions in keeping with Rokitansky–Aschoff sinuses are demonstrated.

The *pearl necklace sign* is attributed to the characteristically curvilinear arrangement of multiple rounded hyperintense intraluminal cavities visualised at T2-weighted MR images. Diffuse, segmental and focal adenomyomatosis exist. Segmental or annular adenomyomatosis appears as limited circumferential gallbladder wall involvement with luminal narrowing, typically within the gallbladder body, which may produce a characteristic hourglass configuration. Focal or localised adenomyomatosis is most common, manifesting as crescentic to rounded gallbladder wall thickening, usually at the fundus. Focal adenomyomatosis may appear as a discrete mass, known as an *adenomyoma*.

Ampullary Tumours

These are tumours that arise from the glandular epithelium of the ampulla of Vater. The ampulla of Vater consists of the bile duct, the main pancreatic duct, the ampulla and the major duodenal papilla surrounded by the sphincter of Oddi.

Ampullary tumours include benign (adenoma) and malignant (carcinoma) forms.

These tumours are usually detected at an early stage because they cause biliary obstruction; therefore, they usually have a better prognosis than their biliary or periampullary counterparts.

Ampullary carcinomas typically are small at the time of diagnosis, and the mass itself can often not be identified at imaging. However, secondary findings such as marked bile duct dilatation, with mild to moderate dilatation of the main pancreatic duct, can usually be seen at imaging. Larger tumours manifest as infiltrative or polypoid masses. Infiltrative lesions appear as an irregularly thickened ductal wall that obliterates the lumen and demonstrates delayed prolonged enhancement, while polypoid masses appear as an intraductal hypodense soft-tissue mass.

Angiomyolipoma

A focal liver lesion that contains various mixtures of adipose tissue, thick-walled arteries and smooth muscle. It is usually asymptomatic; however, bleeding may occur especially in large lesions.

Angiomyolipoma typically presents with high T1-w signal intensity and demonstrates signal drop when fat saturation is applied due to macroscopic fat presence. In cases with minimal macroscopic fat, differential diagnosis from hepatocellular tumours is difficult and biopsy may be performed.

Angiosarcoma

Angiosarcoma is a rare, mesenchymal liver tumour associated with chemical carcinogens such as Thorotrast, vinyl chloride and arsenic ingestion. It affects mostly males, between the sixth and seventh decades.

At the time of diagnosis, usually lung and splenic metastases have occurred. It may present with spontaneous intraperitoneal haemorrhage or with acute liver failure. The most frequent type is diffuse micro- or macronodular.

At CT, most lesions appear hypoattenuating on unenhanced scans and show varied enhancement patterns on multiphasic contrast-enhanced CT.

Imaging features on MRI are of multiple T2-w hyperintense lesions that may be T1-w hyperintense due to haemorrhage and contain fluid–fluid levels. Peripheral and progressive enhancement is noted on post intravenous contrast administration images.

Annular Pancreas

The pancreas develops from a single dorsal and two ventral buds, which appear at 5 weeks of gestation. The two ventral buds fuse rapidly. In the 7th week of gestation, the duodenum expands, and the ventral bud rotates from right to left and fuses with the dorsal bud. The ventral bud forms the inferior portion of the head of the pancreas and the inferior part of the uncinate process, while the dorsal bud forms the body and tail of the pancreas.

Annular pancreas develops due to failure of ventral bud to rotate with duodenum, causing encasement of the duodenum. Annular pancreas can be complete or incomplete. In the complete form, pancreatic parenchyma or annular duct is seen to completely surround the 2nd portion of the duodenum (Fig. 2); in the incomplete form, the annulus does not surround the duodenum completely, giving a “crocodile jaw” appearance.

The reported incidence varies from 1/1,000 to 1/20,000. Two peaks of presentation occur: in the neonatal age, with symptoms of duodenal obstruction, often associated with other congenital abnormalities, and in the adult age, with symptoms of pain or pancreatitis, although up to 33 % cases might be discovered incidentally.

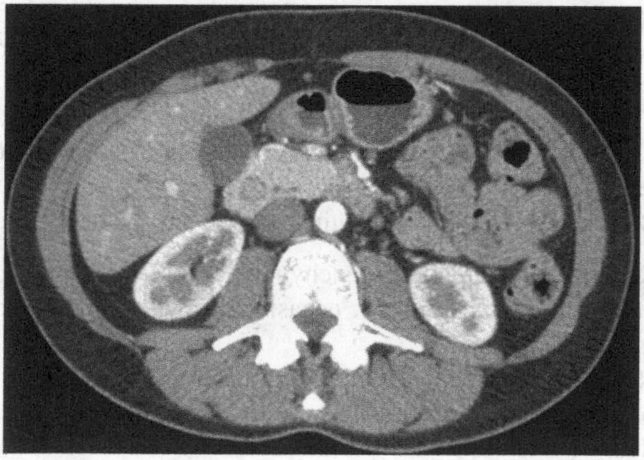

Fig. 2 Annular pancreas: the pancreatic parenchyma surrounds completely the second portion of the duodenum

Autoimmune Pancreatitis

Autoimmune pancreatitis (AIP) is a form of chronic pancreatitis characterised by periductal flogosis, mainly sustained by lymphocytic infiltration, with evolution to fibrosis.

The concept of AIP was first proposed in 1961. Autoimmune pancreatitis classically interests mostly elderly men, although the age range is wide (14–85 years): patients present with chronic pancreatitis without any other cause and with increased serum IgG4. The symptoms are the same as for pancreatic malignancies: fluctuating obstructive jaundice, vague abdominal pain, weight loss, steatorrhoea and diabetes due to a decline in exocrine function.

This form of pancreatitis is called autoimmune because of the association with other autoimmune disease (53 %), the presence of increased IgG or IgG4 and autoantibodies and the dramatic response to steroid treatment.

Imaging has an important role for the diagnosis, to confirm the clinical suspicion, and for the differential diagnosis from pancreatic cancer.

The diagnostic criteria for autoimmune pancreatitis are well defined and include imaging, serology and pathology criteria.

Both below mentioned imaging criteria have to be fulfilled:

1. Regarding pancreatic parenchyma: Diffuse/segmental/focal enlargement of the gland, occasionally with a mass and/or hypoattenuating rim
2. Regarding pancreaticobiliary ducts: Diffuse/segmental/focal pancreatic ductal narrowing, often with stenosis of the bile duct

Three different patterns are recognised at imaging: focal, diffuse or multifocal involvement of the pancreas.

At CT, AIP appears as a solid hypodense lesion, hypovascular in the pancreatic phase, with progressive enhancement in the venous and delayed phases.

At MRI, AIP appears slightly hyperintense on T2-weighted images and hypointense on T1 fat-saturated images (Fig. 3). After Gd administration, AIP appears hypovascular in the pancreatic phase, with progressive enhancement in the venous

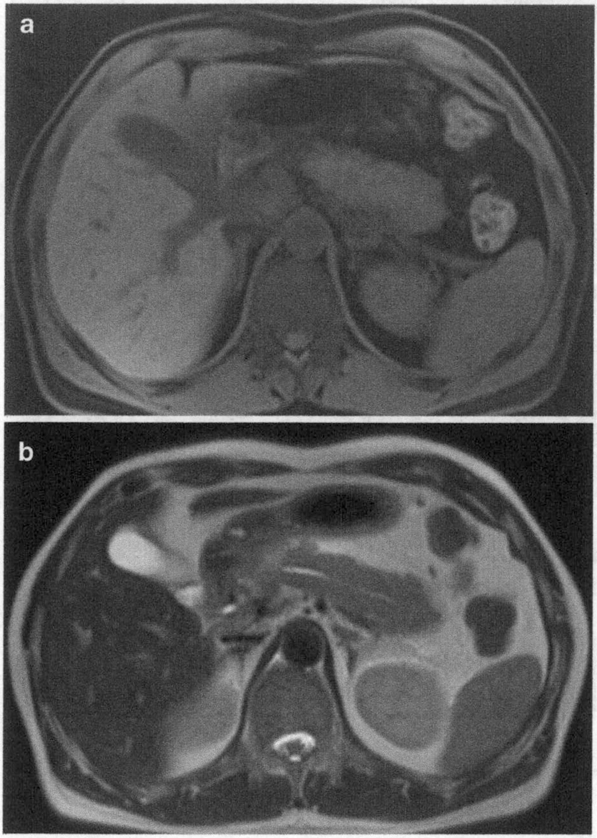

Fig. 3 Autoimmune pancreatitis. The pancreas is enlarged and appears hypointense on T1 fat-saturated image (**a**) and slightly hyperintense on T2-weighted image (**b**). MRCP shows a segmental stenosis of the main pancreatic duct (**c**). After Gd administration, the parenchyma is hypovascular in the pancreatic phase (**d**), with progressive enhancement in the venous (**e**) and delayed (**f**) phases

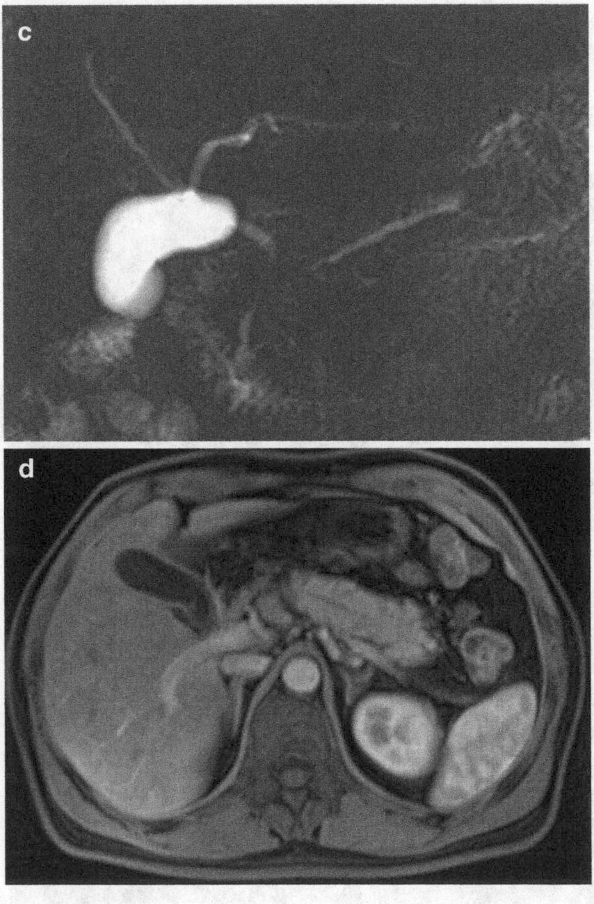

Fig. 3 (continued)

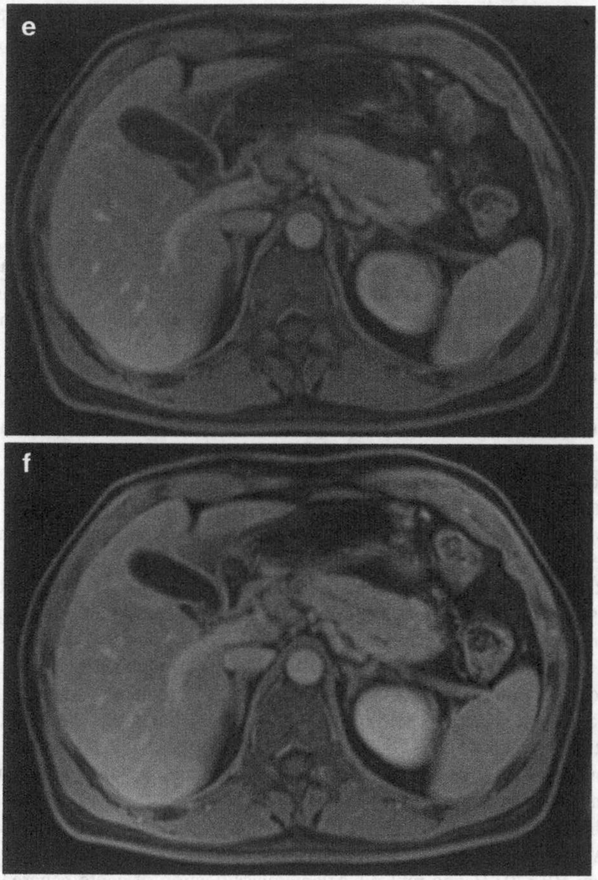

Fig. 3 (continued)

phase. At DWI, AIP shows restricted diffusion. MRCP usually shows stenosis of the main pancreatic duct, which is overcome after administration of secretin (duct-penetrating sign).

Suggested Reading

Banks PA, Bollen TL, Dervenis C et al; Acute Pancreatitis Classification Working Group (2013) Classification of acute pancreatiti--012: revision of the Atlanta classification and definitions by international consensus. Gut 62(1):102–11.

Boscak AR, Al-Hawary M, Ramsburgh SR (2006) Best cases from the AFIP: Adenomyomatosis of the gallbladder. Radiographics 26(3):941–6

Brennan DD, Zamboni GA, Raptopoulos VD et al (2007) Comprehensive preoperative assessment of pancreatic adenocarcinoma with 64-section volumetric CT. Radiographics 27(6):1653–66.

Ichikawa T, Erturk SM, Motosugi U et al (2007) High-b value diffusion-weighted MRI for detecting pancreatic adenocarcinoma: preliminary results. AJR Am J Roentgenol 188(2):409–414

Ichikawa T, Sou H, Araki T et al (2001) Duct-penetrating sign at MRCP: usefulness for differentiating inflammatory pancreatic mass from pancreatic carcinomas. Radiology 221(1):107–16.

Kim JH, Park SH, Yu ES et al (2010) Visually isoattenuating pancreatic adenocarcinoma at dynamic-enhanced CT: frequency, clinical and pathologic characteristics, and diagnosis at imaging examinations. Radiology 257(1):87–96

Sahani DV, Kalva SP, Farrell J et al (2004) Autoimmune pancreatitis: imaging features. Radiology 233 (2): 345–52

Sandrasegaran K, Patel A, Fogel EL et al (2009) Annular pancreas in adults. AJR Am J Roentgenol 193(2):455–60.

Thoeni RF (2012) The revised Atlanta classification of acute pancreatitis: its importance for the radiologist and its effect on treatment. Radiology 262(3):751–64.

B

Biliary Cystadenoma/Cystadenocarcinoma

Biliary cystadenoma is a rare benign cystic hepatic neoplasm with premalignant potential. Biliary cystadenocarcinoma is its malignant counterpart. These tumours originate in the bile ducts and are lined by mucin-secreting epithelium.

Biliary cystadenomas occur predominantly in middle-aged patients, with a female prevalence.

The clinical symptoms are non-specific. It appears as a unilocular or, more commonly, multilocular cystic intrahepatic mass as large as 30 cm. The cyst wall is well defined and enhances after administration of contrast agent. The cyst content has fluid attenuation and is typically hypointense on T1-weighted images and hyperintense on T2-weighted images. Depending on the type of fluid content (e.g. mucin, blood, bile), however, the signal intensity can vary. Cystadenomas occasionally have fine septal calcifications, while cystadenocarcinomas have thick and coarse calcifications. Cystadenocarcinomas may show mural nodules or papillary intraluminal projections.

G. Zamboni, S. Gourtsoyianni, *MDCT and MRI of the Liver, Bile Ducts and Pancreas*, A-Z Notes in Radiological Practice and Reporting, DOI 10.1007/978-88-470-5720-3_2,

Biliary Hamartomas (von Meyenburg Complex)

Biliary hamartomas are benign cystic malformations of the biliary tree. They present as multiple, small, measuring 0.5–1.5 cm in diameter, nonenhancing lesions through both liver lobes, usually in the subcapsular area. On T1-w images these are hypointense, while on T2-w images these are hyperintense, slightly less than simple cysts. Biliary hamartomas may show peripheral enhancement in all phases post IV contrast administration; mural nodule enhancement has also been reported corresponding to an endocystic polypoid projection made of conjunctive septa. These lesions do not appear to communicate with the biliary tree and tend not to grow with time.

Biloma

A biloma is an extrabiliary collection of bile, either intrahepatic or extrahepatic. Bilomas can be spontaneous and post-traumatic or occur as a complication of surgery or percutaneous interventions. Most bilomas develop in the right upper quadrant (70 %), while only 30 % in the left upper quadrant. Bilomas may wall off, or the active bile leakage may continue.

On CT, the bilious fluid appears hypodense, with water-like attenuation.

At MRI the fluid has variable signal intensity on T1-weighted images and appears hyperintense on T2-weighted images, similar to the signal intensity of bile in the gallbladder.

If the diagnosis of biloma is unclear, biliary-excretion MRI agents can be used: a delayed acquisition can show the leak site and confirm the diagnosis.

Budd–Chiari Syndrome

Budd–Chiari syndrome is a rare, venous occlusive disorder, often idiopathic, with most known causes being coagulation disorders, pregnancy, oral contraceptives, infection and tumour thrombus.

Acute, subacute and chronic stages can be distinguished by imaging.

In acute Budd–Chiari syndrome, the liver exhibits patchy, decreased peripheral enhancement caused by portal and sinusoidal stasis and stronger enhancement of the central portions of the liver parenchyma. The thrombosed hepatic veins are hypoattenuating, and the inferior vena cava is compressed by the enlarged caudate lobe. Ascites and splenomegaly are usually present.

In subacute or chronic Budd–Chiari syndrome, portosystemic and intrahepatic collateral vessels are found. Contrast-enhanced CT is useful for depicting regions of hypoperfused liver parenchyma.

Portal vein thrombosis can develop as the result of underlying thrombophilia and stagnation of portal flow caused by outflow block.

In chronic Budd–Chiari syndrome, numerous regenerative nodules may be present, which are markedly and homogeneously hyperattenuating on arterial phase images and remain slightly hyperattenuating on portal venous phase. These may be bright on T1-w MR images and predominantly isointense or hypointense relative to the surrounding liver on T2-weighted images.

On T2-weighted MRI images, liver parenchyma demonstrates heterogeneously increased signal intensity in the peripheral portion of the liver. T2*-weighted gradient-echo sequences as well as T1-weighted sequences post-contrast administration should be used to assess absence of flow within hepatic veins and inferior vena cava. Chronic thrombosis of the inferior vena cava may evolve into calcification.

Suggested Reading

Brancatelli G, Vilgrain V, Federle MP et al (2007) Budd-Chiari syndrome: spectrum of imaging findings. AJR Am J Roentgenol 188(2):W168–76.

Tohmé-Noun C, Cazals D, Noun R et al (2008) Multiple biliary hamartomas: magnetic resonance features with histopathologic correlation. Eur Radiol. 18(3):493–9

C

CA 19-9

CA 19-9 is a serum antigen used in the diagnosis and management of hepato-pancreatico-biliary malignancies, although it is non-specific and can rise also in non-malignant conditions such as heavy tea consumption.

CA 19-9>100 U/ml may have a sensitivity of 50 % in diagnosing cholangiocarcinoma, while using an upper limit of normal at 37 U/ml achieves approximately 80 % sensitivity and 90 % specificity for pancreatic adenocarcinoma.

Caroli's Disease

Caroli's disease is an autosomal-recessive congenital disorder comprising of multifocal cystic dilatations of segmental intrahepatic bile ducts. It was first reported by Todd in 1818, but Jacques Caroli in 1958 defined it precisely with the different types.

G. Zamboni, S. Gourtsoyianni, *MDCT and MRI of the Liver, Bile Ducts and Pancreas*, A-Z Notes in Radiological Practice and Reporting, DOI 10.1007/978-88-470-5720-3_3,

The more common form of the disease is associated with periportal fibrosis and may progress to portal hypertension and cirrhosis. The less common "pure" or "simple" form is associated with intrahepatic stones, cholangitis and abscesses. Patients affected by Caroli's disease have an increased risk of developing cholangiocarcinoma (up to 7 % of cases).

The estimated incidence of Caroli's disease is 1 in 1,000,000, with no sex prevalence; more than 80 % of patients are diagnosed before the age of 30 years.

Patients with the most common type of Caroli's disease present with symptoms related to hepatic fibrosis and portal hypertension, while those affected by the pure form present with recurrent attacks of cholangitis.

The characteristic CT appearance is multiple hypoattenuating cystic structures of variable size, which communicate with the biliary system. The "central dot sign" is highly suggestive of Caroli's disease: tiny foci of contrast enhancement within the dilated intrahepatic bile ducts, corresponding to intraluminal portal vein radicles.

On MRI the dilated cystic biliary system appears hypointense on T1-weighted images and hyperintense on T2-weighted images. The *central dot sign* is appreciated also on post-gadolinium MRI images. MRCP demonstrates continuity of the cystic areas with the biliary tree.

Cavernous Transformation of the Portal Vein

Cavernous transformation of the portal vein consists of the formation of venous channels within and around a previously stenosed or occluded portal vein that act as porto-portal collateral vessels.

This cavernous transformation can occur as soon as 6–20 days after the thrombotic event, even if the thrombus is partially recanalised.

In case of portal vein thrombosis, if the portal vein does not recanalise (e.g. in patients with cirrhosis or chronic liver disease), the collateral paracholedochal veins dilate and become serpiginous. These veins drain into the left and right portal branches, or more distally into the liver parenchyma, forming a porto-portal shunt which however is usually insufficient to bypass the entire splenomesenteric inflow, and portal hypertension occurs.

The initial diagnosis is usually made at US, but CT and MRI can confirm it and better depict the anatomy. The most frequent finding is a characteristic beaded appearance (mass of veins) at the porta hepatis, with vessels that enhance in the portal venous phase. Calcifications can be present in the thrombosed portal vein.

Chemoembolisation

Transarterial chemoembolisation (TACE) refers to the administration of chemotherapeutic agents through selective catheterisation of the hepatic arteries. The chemotherapeutic agent can be mixed with iodised oil or adsorbed onto microspheres. The administration is followed by embolisation to stop arterial flow to the lesions. TACE is used most commonly for intermediate-stage HCC but also for hypervascular liver metastases.

The rationale is based on the fact that HCC and liver metastases receive blood supply from the hepatic artery, while the surrounding healthy liver parenchyma receives it from the portal vein. Chemoembolisation offers the ability to expose tumours to high local chemotherapeutic agent concentrations with minimal systemic drug bioavailability.

Cholangiocarcinoma (CCC)

Cholangiocarcinoma is a malignant tumour that may arise at any point of the biliary epithelium from intrahepatic biliary radicals to the ampulla of Vater. The majority of cases are adenocarcinomas. There is a strong association with *Primary sclerosing cholangitis (PSC)*.

Intrahepatic and extrahepatic types exist with intrahepatic further classified as peripheral and perihilar, the latter also known as Klatskin tumour, being the most common type. Less frequently the tumour presents along the common hepatic duct and common bile duct.

Klatskin tumour is further classified as:

Type 1: >2 cm distance to bifurcation
Type 2: <2 cm distance, no involvement of bifurcation
Type 3: involvement of bifurcation
Type 4: involvement of intrahepatic branch ducts

Four different growth patterns have been identified:

(a) Exophytic, where tumour grows outside the bile ducts and forms a mass, characteristic of the peripheral CCC
(b) Infiltrative, along and engulfing the biliary tree, typical for perihilar and extrahepatic type
(c) Polypoid, with intraluminal growth
(d) Combined

Mass-forming cholangiocarcinomas are typically homogeneously hypodense on non-contrast CT and show heterogeneous peripheral enhancement, with enhancement in the delayed phase. Capsular retraction may be present and the bile ducts distal to the mass are typically dilated.

Periductal infiltrating tumours appear as thickening of the periductal parenchyma with altered calibre of the involved duct, which can be narrowed or dilated. There is usually some distal dilatation of the biliary tree.

At MRI, CCC appears hypointense on T1-w and hyperintense on T2-w images and may present with delayed enhancement. A thickened bile duct wall >5 mm is considered suspicious.

Cholangitis

Acute cholangitis occurs due to bacterial infection of the obstructed biliary tree from the GI tract or the portal venous system. Cholangitis is a life-threatening condition if untreated which may also lead to hepatic abscess formation.

Typical imaging findings are thickening of biliary ducts, presenting with mural enhancement as well as irregularity and beading of intrahepatic bile ducts.

Bile duct stenosis may cause chronic or recurrent cholangitis with cholestasis.

Cholecystitis

Ultrasound is the examination of choice for suspected acute cholecystitis with reported sensitivity and specificity >95 %. Imaging findings are (a) thickened gallbladder wall > 3 mm, (b) presence of pericholecystic fluid, as well as (c) tenderness over GB during examination, the so-called sonographic Murphy's sign. Gallstones are identified in calculous cholecystitis.

CT is better in demonstrating pericholecystic inflammatory changes and complications of acute cholecystitis.

Gangrenous cholecystitis is a serious complication of acute cholecystitis. It is the result of marked distension of the gallbladder causing increased tension in the gallbladder wall. Associated inflammation leads to ischemic necrosis of the wall, with or without associated cystic artery thrombosis. It is more common in men and in patients with coexisting cardiovascular disease and leucocytosis, and on imaging, intramural gas is demonstrated.

In *chronic cholecystitis*, the gallbladder appears small and contracted, with irregular and thickened wall, which enhances less intensely than in acute cholecystitis. Gallstones are identified.

Choledochal Cysts

Choledochal cysts are congenital anomalies of the bile ducts, consisting of cystic dilatations of the extrahepatic biliary tree, the intrahepatic biliary radicles or both.

Choledochal cysts are rare, with an incidence of 1:100,000–150,000 and a female prevalence of 3–4:1. Although the condition may be discovered in the adult age, most cases are diagnosed during infancy or childhood, and approximately 67 % of patients present with signs or symptoms related to the cyst before the age of 10 years.

Choledochal cysts are usually classified according to the classification devised by Todani et al. This classification recognises 5 main types and several subtypes:

- Type I—most common form (80–90 %), can present in utero
  - Ia—dilatation of the entire extrahepatic bile duct
  - Ib—segmental dilatation of the extrahepatic bile duct
  - Ic—dilatation of the common bile duct portion of the extrahepatic bile duct
- Type II—true diverticulum from the extrahepatic bile duct
- Type III—dilatation of the extrahepatic bile duct within the duodenal wall (choledochocele)

- Type IV—the second most common form
  - IVa—cysts involving both intra- and extrahepatic ducts
  - IVb—multiple dilatations/cysts of extrahepatic ducts only
- Type V—multiple dilatations/cysts of intrahepatic ducts only (Caroli's disease)

The diagnosis is made when a cystic dilatation is identified which communicates with the bile duct and is distinct from the gallbladder.

CT and MRI can both depict the anatomy and allow a diagnosis. The use of CT cholangiography has been proposed to demonstrate communication between the cyst and the biliary system.

The two most frequent complications of choledochal cysts are stone formation and malignancy.

Cholangiocarcinoma is the most feared complication, with a reported incidence of 9–28 %.

Choledocholithiasis

Choledocholithiasis is the presence of calculi within the common bile duct that most commonly have migrated from the gallbladder. In most cases it is symptomatic.

MRCP examination is considered the non-invasive examination of choice to rule out the presence of bile duct calculi, which are identified as filling defects within the high T2-w signal intensity bile content of the duct.

Chronic Pancreatitis

Chronic pancreatitis is a continuing inflammatory process of the pancreas characterised by progressive parenchyma destruction with exocrine and endocrine insufficiency.

The most easily identified findings are atrophy and alterations in size, which occur in the advanced stages of the disease.

The most significant findings for the diagnosis are intraductal calcifications, pancreatic duct dilatation (i.e. calibre >3 mm) and pseudocysts.

The presence of calcifications is the most important diagnostic criterion, according to the Japan Pancreas Society, and is pathognomonic for chronic pancreatitis.

CT is usually the first modality used in the assessment of patients with chronic pancreatitis, but in the early phases, CT may not show significant findings. CT findings of chronic pancreatitis include intraductal and parenchymal calcifications, pancreatic duct dilatation and parenchymal atrophy (Fig. 1).

MRI with MRCP and S-MRCP are the imaging modality of choice for the diagnosis, as they allow to recognise the parenchymal and ductal changes typical of early chronic pancreatitis. MRI will show multiple slight strictures and/or parietal irregularities of the main pancreatic duct.

Secretin-MRCP allows better evaluation of the MPD calibre and its functional changes, the duodenal filling, the presence of branch-duct dilation and the presence of “acinar filling”.

MRCP criteria for disease identification include abnormal ductal response to secretin, progressive enhancement of the pancreatic parenchyma related to a loss of ductal or parenchymal compliance (so-called acinar filling), characteristic side-branch involvement and changes in gadolinium uptake (decreased and heterogeneous early enhancement and delayed enhancement).

Diffusion-weighted imaging coupled with secretin administration can aid in the diagnosis of chronic pancreatitis: a delayed peak ADC or a very low baseline ADC coupled with no response to secretin is useful for the diagnosis.

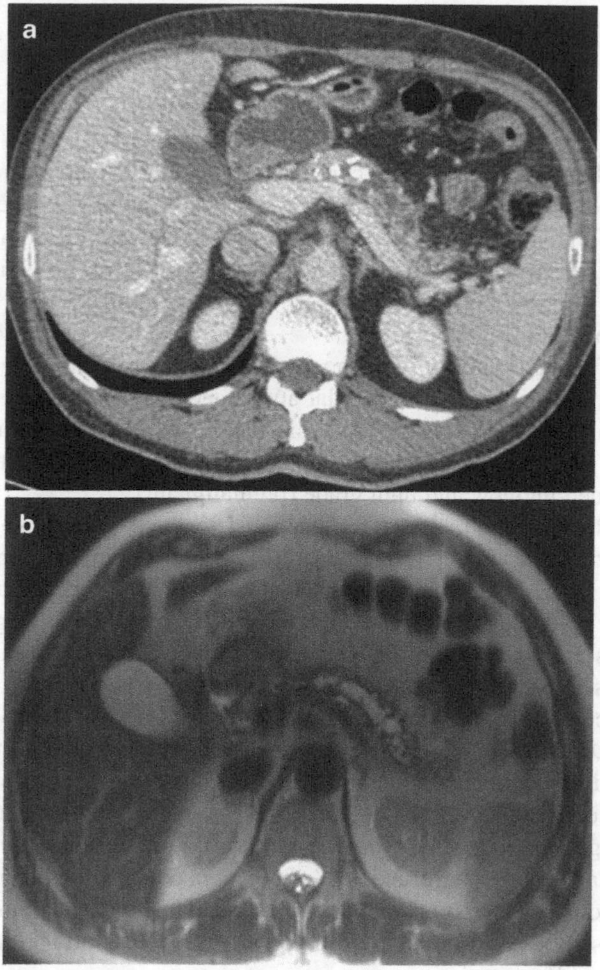

Fig. 1 Chronic pancreatitis. Axial venous phase CT image shows calcific calculi in the lumen of the main pancreatic duct, with upstream ductal dilatation and parenchymal atrophy (**a**). Axial T2-weighted MR image shows the tortuous dilated main pancreatic duct and multiple dilated side branches (**b**)

Cirrhosis

- Regenerative Nodule
- Dysplastic Nodule

Hepatic cirrhosis is a chronic inflammatory liver disorder pathologically defined by extensive fibrosis, nodular regeneration and architectural distortion of the parenchyma including a nodular surface contour, caudate lobe hyperplasia, right liver lobe atrophy, left liver lobe hypertrophy and prominent fat in the hepatic hilum.

The vast majority of cirrhosis-related nodules exhibit regenerative changes without cellular atypia and are known as regenerative nodules (RNs), while a minority have dysplastic features and are known as dysplastic nodules (DNs); these are further divided into low and high grade (premalignant).

RNs are small, <2 cm, homogenous, nonencapsulated, iso- or hypointense on T1-weighted and T2-weighted images. Iron-containing nodules, present in haemochromatosis, appear markedly hypointense on T2-weighted and T2*-weighted images. RNs are isointense to the surrounding liver parenchyma in all phases as well as in the hepatobiliary phase post hepatocyte specific IV contrast administration.

DNs are T1-w iso- to hyperintense, in case of glycogen or lipid content. Lipid-containing nodules display signal loss on out-of-phase GRE images. In post IV contrast administration images, these are hyperintense on arterial phase/isointense on portal venous phase and late phase or isointense on arterial/ hypointense on portal venous/late phase, while on hepatobiliary phase, these are isointense to hyperintense (related to their cellular differentiation).

Any T2-w hyperintensity within the nodules, or nodule within nodule configuration, should be considered a sign of atypia or early sign of neoplastic degeneration.

Clonorchiasis

Clonorchiasis is a trematodiasis caused by chronic infestation by *Clonorchis sinensis* and can lead to recurrent pyogenic cholangitis, biliary strictures and cholangiocarcinoma. Infection occurs after ingestion of infected raw flesh of freshwater fish.

Signs and symptoms are usually mild and non-specific; heavy infestation can result in obstructive jaundice.

CT typically shows diffuse dilatation of the peripheral intrahepatic bile ducts, without dilation of the larger bile ducts or extrahepatic ducts: these findings are considered to be the pathognomonic for clonorchiasis; however they persist when the infection is cured.

MR imaging can show the characteristic diffuse, mild dilation of the small peripheral intrahepatic bile ducts. The presence of "too many intrahepatic ducts" at MRCP has been described in 62 % of patients with clonorchiasis. MRI can show periductal enhancement. The flukes can be seen as elliptical, irregular-shaped hypointense filling defects on T2-weighted images and MRCP.

Suggested Reading

Choi BI, Kim TK, Han JK (1998) MRI of clonorchiasis and cholangiocarcinoma. J Magn Reson Imaging 8(2):359–66.

Gallego C, Velasco M, Marcuello P et al (2002) Congenital and acquired anomalies of the portal venous system. Radiographics 22(1):141–59.

Hanna RF, Aguirre DA, Kased N et al (2008) Cirrhosis-associated hepatocellular nodules: correlation of histopathologic and MR imaging features. Radiographics 28(3):747–69.

Homma T, Harada H, Koizumi M (1997) Diagnostic criteria for chronic pancreatitis by the Japan Pancreas Society. Pancreas 15(1):14–5.

Jeong YY, Kang HK, Kim JW et al (2004) MR imaging findings of clonorchiasis. Korean J Radiol. 5(1):25–30.

Kim OH, Chung HJ, Choi BG (1995) Imaging of the choledochal cyst. Radiographics. 15(1):69–88.

Lim JH (1990) Radiologic findings of clonorchiasis. AJR Am J Roentgenol 155 (5): 1001–8.

Vachha B, Sun MR, Siewert B et al (2011) Cystic Lesions of the Liver. AJR Am J Roentgenol 196: W355–W366.

Yu J, Turner MA, Fulcher AS et al (2006) Congenital anomalies and normal variants of the pancreaticobiliary tract and the pancreas in adults: part 1, Biliary tract. AJR Am J Roentgenol 187 (6): 1536–43

D

Diffusion-Weighted Imaging (Focal Liver Lesions)

Diffusion-weighted MR imaging (DW MRI) enables qualitative, by visual assessment, and quantitative assessment of tissue diffusivity, by means of apparent diffusion coefficient (ADC) measurements, without the use of gadolinium chelates, which makes it a highly attractive technique, particularly in patients at risk for nephrogenic systemic fibrosis.

DW MRI is used with great success for the detection and characterisation of focal liver lesions and their differentiation (benign from malignant) in combination with conventional MR sequences. It also provides information regarding tumour treatment response assessment by monitoring change in ADC values of lesions (expressed in 10^{-3} mm^2/s).

Hypercellular tissues, such as tumours or abscesses, demonstrate restricted diffusion (high signal intensity) on higher b value images and lower ADC values. On the other hand, cystic or necrotic lesions show a greater degree of signal attenuation, demonstrating low signal intensity on higher *b* value diffusion

G. Zamboni, S. Gourtsoyianni, *MDCT and MRI of the Liver, Bile Ducts and Pancreas*, A-Z Notes in Radiological Practice and Reporting, DOI 10.1007/978-88-470-5720-3_4,

images, and return higher ADC values. One has to keep in mind that lesions may appear to show restricted diffusion due to their long T2-relaxation time as well, when correlating high b value images with corresponding ADC map (lesions show high signal intensity on both). This phenomenon is called T2 shine-through and may be observed in the normal gallbladder, cystic lesions and haemangiomas (pathognomonic). Generally ADC values tend to be lower than those of normal liver parenchyma in malignant tumours and higher in benign liver lesions.

Dorsal Agenesis of the Pancreas

Partial agenesis of the pancreas is an extremely rare malformation, which more often involves the dorsal pancreas. It results from an embryological failure of the dorsal pancreatic bud to form the body and tail of the pancreas. Dorsal agenesis can be isolated or part of heterotaxia syndromes.

In the complete form, the neck, body and tail of the pancreas, the duct of Santorini and the minor duodenal papilla are all absent.

In the partial form, the size of the body of the pancreas varies, there is a remnant of the duct of Santorini, and the minor duodenal papilla is present.

Most patients are asymptomatic and the diagnosis is incidental. The diagnosis is suggested when imaging does not show any pancreatic tissue ventral to the splenic vein. This situation goes into differential diagnosis with pancreatic lipomatosis, where the pancreas is substituted by fat. In the case of agenesis, MRCP and ERCP will not show any ductal structures, which are present in case of lipomatosis.

Double Duct Sign

The double duct sign consists in the presence of simultaneous dilatation of the common bile duct and the main pancreatic duct, highly suggestive for the presence of a pancreatic head malignancy.

It is an anatomical sign which can be seen on all modalities (MRI, CT, US, ERCP).

The two most common causes of the double duct sign are carcinoma of the head of the pancreas and ampullary carcinoma. However, this sign can be present also in cholangiocarcinoma of the distal common bile duct, metastases or lymphoma, and also in benign conditions such as ampullary stenosis and chronic pancreatitis.

Duct-Penetrating Sign

This is a valuable sign for the differential diagnosis between benign and malignant strictures of the main pancreatic duct.

The "duct-penetrating sign" on MRCP images—a smoothly stenotic or normal main pancreatic duct penetrating into a mass—has high sensitivity and specificity (100 %) in the diagnosis of benign stricture.

Suggested Reading

Ahualli J (2007) The double duct sign. Radiology 244(1):314–5.
Gourtsoyianni S, Papanikolaou N, Yarmenitis S et al (2008) Respiratory gated diffusion-weighted imaging of the liver: value of apparent diffusion coefficient measurements in the differentiation between most

commonly encountered benign and malignant focal liver lesions. Eur Radiol 18(3):486–92
Ichikawa T, Sou H, Araki T et al (2001) Duct-penetrating sign at MRCP: usefulness for differentiating inflammatory pancreatic mass from pancreatic carcinomas. Radiology 221(1):107–16.
Taouli B, Koh DM (2010) Diffusion-weighted MR imaging of the liver. Radiology 254(1):47–66.

E

Echinococcal Cyst (Hydatid Cyst)

It is a parasitic infection with *Echinococcus granulosus*. The infection occurs by direct contact with a dog (which is the final host, while sheep and cattle are the intermediate hosts) or via contaminated water or food. Embryos migrate through the intestinal mucosa and reach the liver through the portal vein. Cysts formed in the liver may grow 2–3 cm per year. When small, these are identical to simple liver cysts, while larger cysts form daughter cysts and membranes that can slough off or rupture. Pathognomonic imaging features are presence of calcifications seen in the capsule, best appreciated on CT (Fig. 1), or evidence of a floating membrane within ruptured lamellae (Fig. 2). The most severe complication is cyst rupture within the abdominal cavity.

G. Zamboni, S. Gourtsoyianni, *MDCT and MRI of the Liver, Bile Ducts and Pancreas*, A-Z Notes in Radiological Practice and Reporting, DOI 10.1007/978-88-470-5720-3_5,

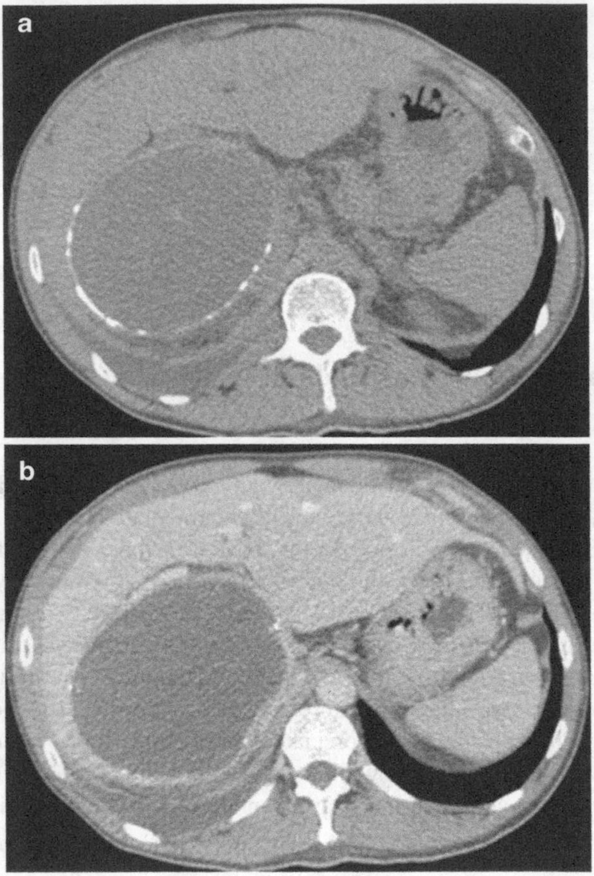

Fig. 1 Echinococcal cyst. Unenhanced (**a**) and venous phase (**b**) CT images show a large cystic lesion in the right liver lobe, with a thick enhancing wall with calcifications. Fluid content is hyperintense on coronal T2-w MRI (**c**). Wall enhancement is well depicted also in arterial post-Gd MRI (**d**)

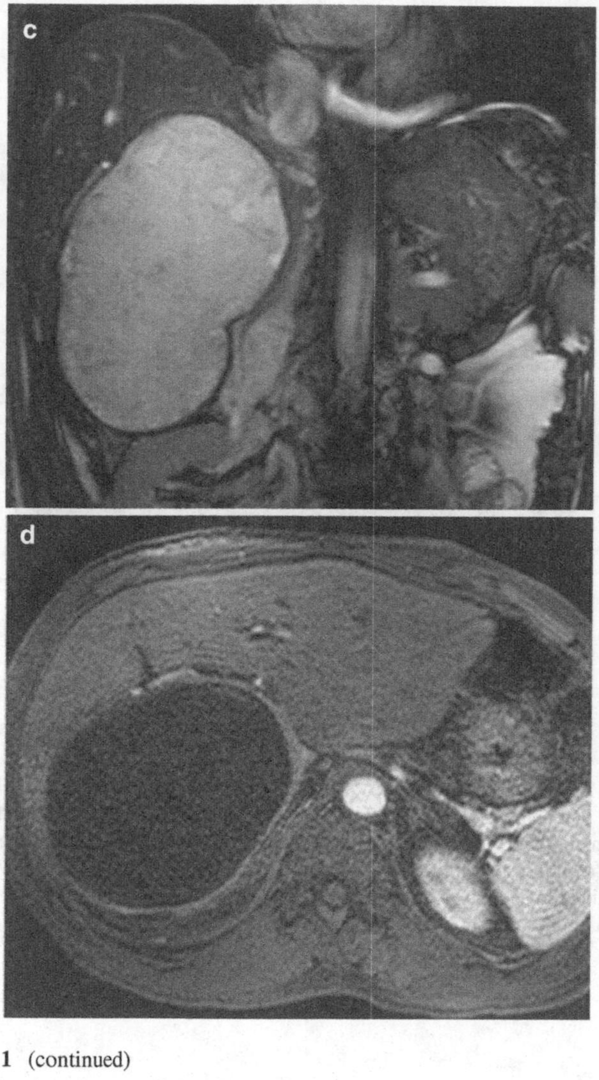

Fig. 1 (continued)

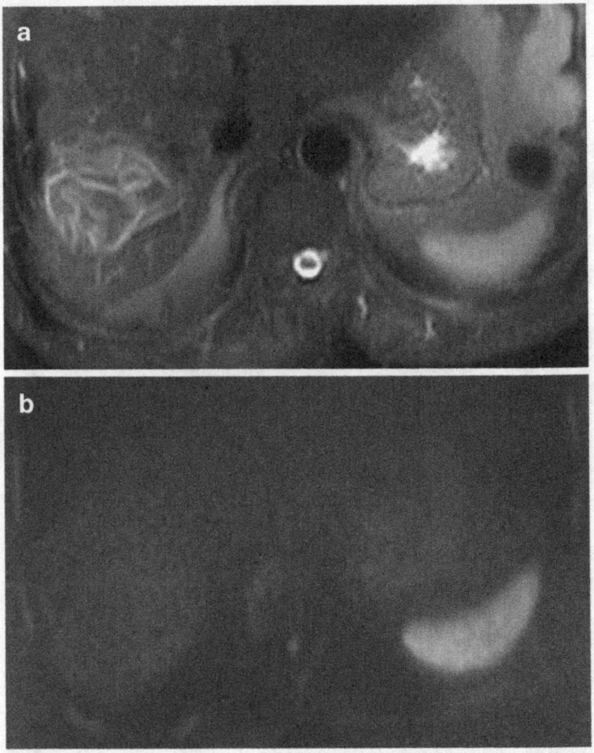

Fig. 2 Echinococcal cyst. Focal liver lesion in segment 7 of the right liver lobe that demonstrates T2-w hyperintense linear bands suggestive of floating membrane within ruptured lamellae (**a**). Note that this is a cystic lesion that demonstrates free diffusion, low signal intensity on highest b value obtained images (**b**) and high signal intensity on corresponding ADC map (**c**) and does not show any abnormal contrast uptake (**d**)

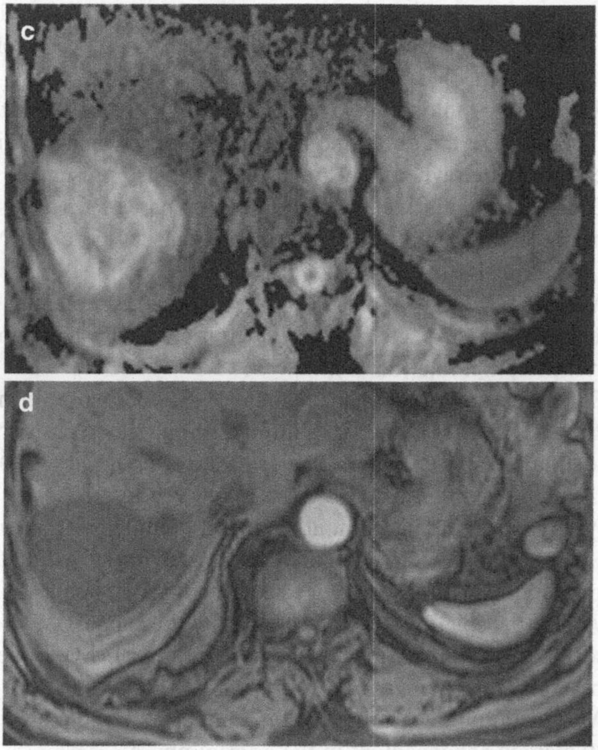

Fig. 2 (continued)

Endocrine Tumours of the Pancreas

Endocrine tumours of the pancreas arise from the pancreatic islet cells and include a number of distinct tumours that match the cell type of origin.

Endocrine tumours can be classified as hyperfunctioning or nonfunctioning based on the synthesis and secretion of functioning hormones. Hyperfunctioning tumours include insulinomas and gastrinomas, the two most common functioning tumours, and more rare entities such as glucagonoma, somatostatinoma and VIPoma.

Functioning tumours are usually diagnosed at an earlier stage and smaller size than nonfunctioning tumours, which are diagnosed more often when liver metastases are also present.

Endocrine tumours can be sporadic or part of certain syndromes, including multiple endocrine neoplasia type 1 (MEN 1) and von Hippel–Lindau (VHL) disease.

Although MDCT is usually the first choice imaging for patients with a suspected endocrine tumour, MRI has similar overall detection rate (85 %).

Endocrine tumours appear isodense or hyperdense on noncontrast CT. After contrast administration, most commonly these tumours appear hypervascular in the arterial phase (90 %) and remain hyperdense or isodense in the venous phase.

Pancreatic endocrine tumours appear hypointense to the normal parenchyma on T1-weighted images, with or without fat suppression. Fat-suppressed T1-weighted GRE images yield very high conspicuity for the tumour, which appears hypointense. On T2-weighted images, the tumour appears hyperintense to the normal parenchyma.

After gadolinium administration, endocrine tumours usually show marked enhancement in the arterial phase.

Suggested Reading

Megibow AJ (2012) Unusual solid pancreatic tumors. Radiol Clin North Am. 50(3):499–51

F

Fibrocystic Liver Diseases

Fibrocystic liver diseases, or ductal plate malformations, are a group of congenital diseases resulting from abnormal embryogenesis of the biliary ductal system.

The abnormalities include choledochal cyst, Caroli's disease and Caroli's syndrome, adult autosomal dominant polycystic liver disease and biliary hamartoma.

Fibrolamellar Carcinoma (FLC)

Fibrolamellar carcinoma is a rare liver malignancy, presenting in a younger population of patients without evidence of hepatitis or cirrhosis. It is a well-defined, nonencapsulated, large, solitary lesion with expansile growth pattern and lobulated margins. It may contain calcifications and present with a central scar that is hypointense on T1-w images, hypo/hyperintense on T2-w images and hypovascular on equilibrium phase. Differential diagnosis has to be made from FNH. Fibrolamellar carcinoma

G. Zamboni, S. Gourtsoyianni, *MDCT and MRI of the Liver, Bile Ducts and Pancreas*, A-Z Notes in Radiological Practice and Reporting, DOI 10.1007/978-88-470-5720-3_6,

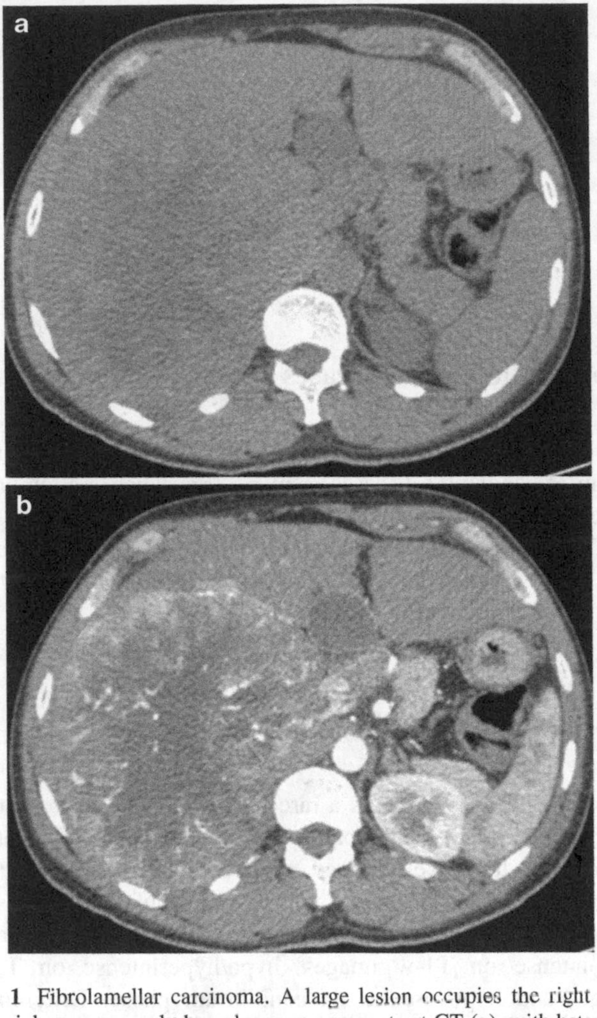

Fig. 1 Fibrolamellar carcinoma. A large lesion occupies the right liver lobe, inhomogeneously hypodense on non-contrast CT (**a**), with heterogeneous arterial enhancement (**b**), and isodense on venous (**c**) and delayed-phase images (**d**)

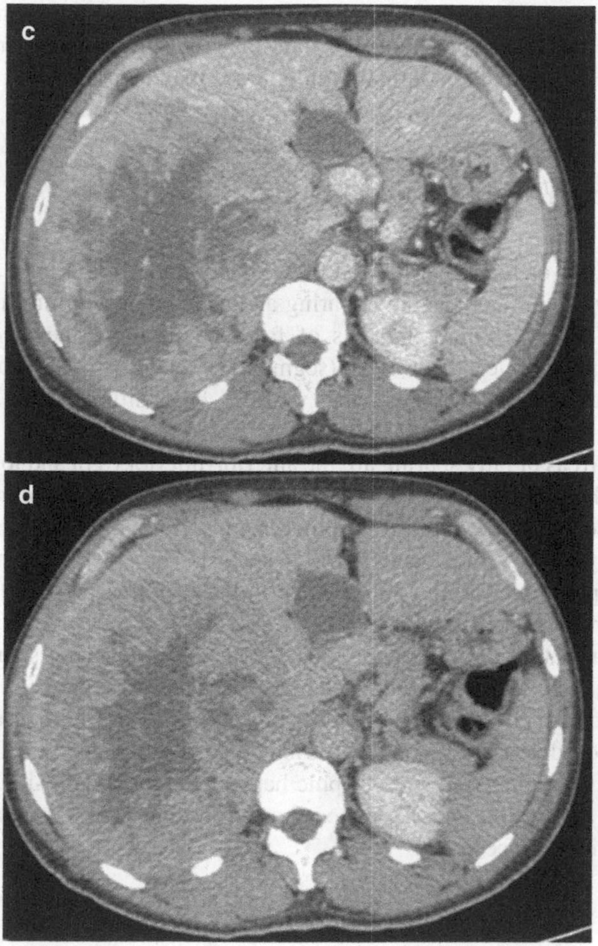

Fig. 1 (continued)

demonstrates heterogeneous arterial enhancement with isointensity or slight persistent hyperintensity in the delayed phase due to abundant fibrous tissue within the lesion (Fig. 1).

With hepatocyte-specific contrast agents, FLC does not show significant enhancement and thus may be differentiated from FNH. Regional abdominal lymph nodes may be present.

Focal Fatty Change (Liver)

Uneven or focal distribution of fat is common in the liver and may present both as fatty sparing and as focal fatty infiltration.

The most common areas of fat deposition are the medial segment of left liver lobe (segment IV), close to the portal bifurcation and around the vessels, best differentiated by chemical shift imaging.

Areas of fatty sparing are the anterior-inferior right and lower medial left IVb segments in the vicinity of the gallbladder, as these areas have a different blood supply from aberrant vessels carrying systemic venous blood such as the inferior vein of Sappey (falciform ligament), peribiliary venous system and aberrant gastric drainage veins.

In patients with hepatic steatosis, a perilesional fat-sparing ring may be seen surrounding metastases and vascularised liver lesions such as haemangiomas, presenting as a bright rim on opposed-phase T1 images, attributed to decreased portal flow due to compressed and atrophic hepatocyte cords with sinusoidal congestion and presence of arterioportal perfusion abnormalities, respectively.

Nodular fatty changes lack T2-w hyperintensity and arterial hypervascularity. Focal fatty sparing is iso- or hypointense on in-phase T1-weighted images and hyperintense on opposed-phase images, while focal fatty infiltration or focal steatosis is iso- to hyperintense on in-phase T1-w images and hypointense on opposed-phase images.

Focal Nodular Hyperplasia (FNH)

FNH occurs in about 1 % of the population and is a benign focal liver lesion consisting of normal liver components in an abnormal organised pattern with blind ductules that do not lead to larger bile ducts. In 60–70 % a central stellate scar and fibrous septa are present. The differential diagnosis for lesions with a central scar includes fibrolamellar HCC, adenoma and intrahepatic CCC. FNH rarely grows or bleeds.

On dynamic extracellular contrast agent MR imaging, it shows strong enhancement in the arterial phase and becomes isointense to surrounding liver parenchyma on portal venous phase (Fig. 2).

Use of hepatocyte-specific contrast agents increases the diagnostic confidence, as FNH demonstrates slow biliary excretion compared to the surrounding normal liver parenchyma and thus remains hyperintense in the hepatobiliary phase.

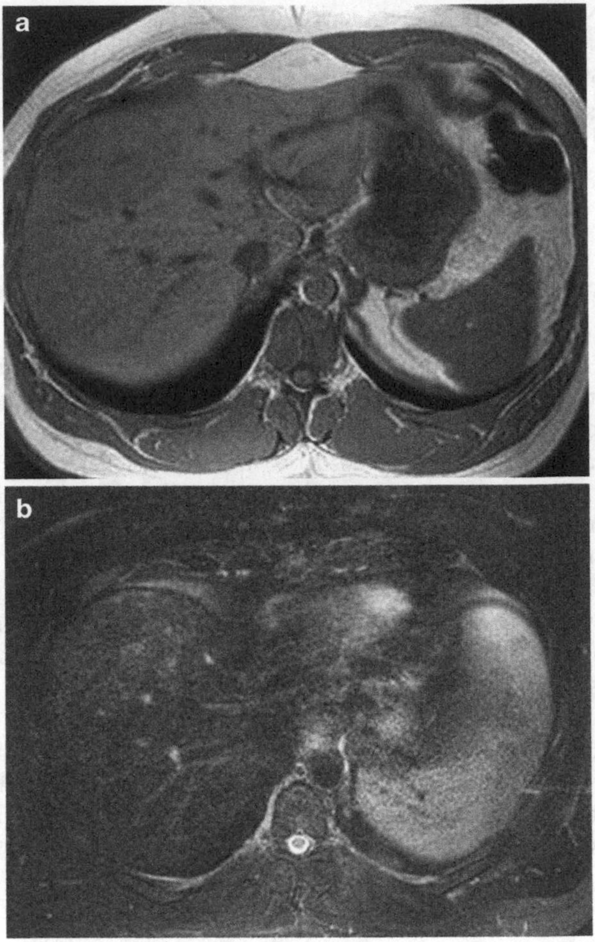

Fig. 2 FNH: incidental focal liver lesion with subcapsular location in segment IVa in a 32-year-old male. Lesion is slightly hypointense on T1-w (**a**) and slightly hyperintense on T2-w (**b**), is avidly enhancing on arterial phase apart from small central scar area (**c**) and retains contrast uptake on hepatocyte-specific contrast phase after Gd-EOB-DTPA administration (**d**)

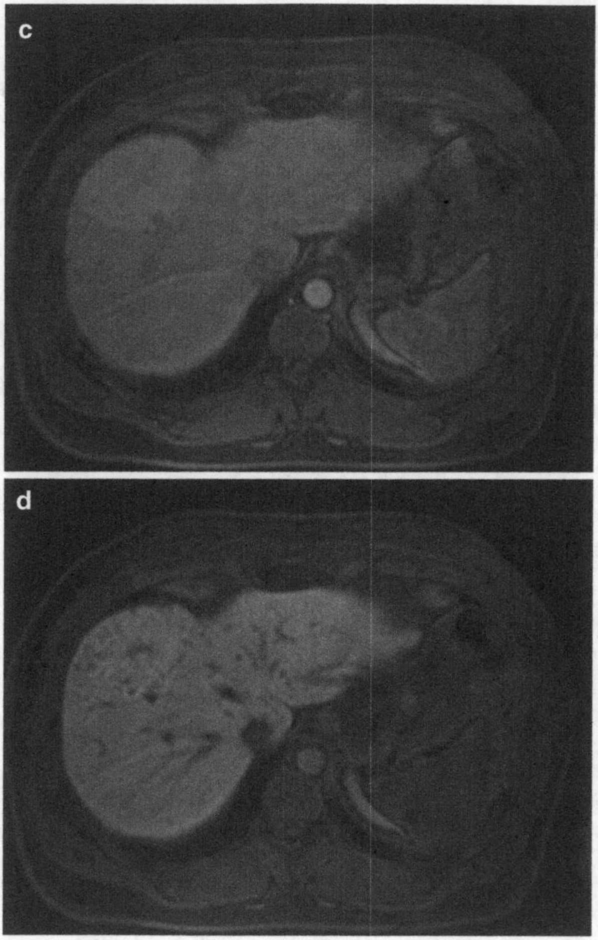

Fig. 2 (continued)

Suggested Reading

Hamrick-Turner JE, Shipkey FH, Cranston PE (1994) Fibrolamellar hepatocellular carcinoma: MR appearance mimicking focal nodular hyperplasia. J Comput Assist Tomogr. 18(2):301–4

Marin D, Iannaccone R, Laghi A, et al (2007) Focal nodular hyperplasia: intraindividual comparison of dynamic gadobenate dimeglumine- and ferucarbotran-enhanced magnetic resonance imaging. J Magn Reson Imaging 25(4):775–82

Martí-Bonmatí L, Peñaloza F, Villarreal E et al (2005) Nonspecificity of the fat-sparing ring surrounding focal liver lesion at MR imaging. Acad Radiol. 12(12):1551–6

Venkatanarasimha N, Thomas R, Armstrong EM et al (2011) Imaging features of ductal plate malformations in adults. Clin Radiol 66(11): 1086–93.

G

Gallbladder Adenocarcinoma

Related to long-standing chronic calculous cholecystitis, porcelain gallbladder, a condition of partial/complete gallbladder wall calcification associated with chronic inflammation, as well as PSC.

Two distinctive types are described: polypoid and infiltrative. The gallbladder fundus is the most common site, which may be confused with the fundal variant of adenomyoma.

Gallbladder adenocarcinoma is usually asymptomatic until the late stage, when the large, infiltrating mass causes obstructive jaundice due to external compression of the common bile duct.

On CT it is usually identified as focal or diffuse mural thickening demonstrating variable enhancement and may also be obscuring the gallbladder and/or involve the adjacent liver parenchyma, hepatic flexure and regional lymph nodes, causing biliary obstruction and giving haematogenous metastases.

G. Zamboni, S. Gourtsoyianni, *MDCT and MRI of the Liver, Bile Ducts and Pancreas*, A-Z Notes in Radiological Practice and Reporting, DOI 10.1007/978-88-470-5720-3_7,

Gallbladder Polyp

Adenomatous and hyperplastic polyps are incidental findings on US examination. The majority are not of clinical significance; however due to the remote possibility of early GB malignancy, polyps > 1 cm should be considered suspicious. Gallbladder polyps may be differentiated from small gallbladder calculi due to lack of posterior acoustic shadow and the fact that these are not mobile upon changing patient's position (left lateral decubitus, upright) during US examination.

Gallstones

Seventy to eighty percent of gallstones are cholesterol stones with pigment, while mixed and calcium carbonate calculi comprise the remainder. Ultrasound is the imaging modality of choice for suspected gallstones. These present as echogenic intraluminal structures with associated posterior acoustic shadow. On CT gallstones may present as calcified round structures or as hypodense intraluminal lesions, characteristic of cholesterol stones. At MRI gallstones appear as filling defects within the high T2-w signal intensity bile contained in the gallbladder.

Suggested Reading

Catalano OA, Sahani DV, Kalva SP et al (2008) MR imaging of the gallbladder: a pictorial essay. Radiographics 28(1):135–55

H

Haemangioendothelioma, Epithelioid

Hepatic epithelioid haemangioendothelioma (HEHE) is a rare, malignant, vascular tumour which originates from endothelial cells and is more common among women. Its histologic appearance and behaviour range between haemangioma and haemangiosarcoma.

HEHE is known to occur in individuals of all ages, and no definitive etiological factor has been clearly identified. Its rarity and non-specific symptoms make the diagnosis of this entity very challenging, with the majority of cases being misdiagnosed.

There are two subtypes: the nodular, present in early stages, characterised by multifocal nodules, and the diffuse subtype at later stages when nodules grow and eventually coalesce, forming large confluent masses preferentially involving the periphery of the liver.

There is great heterogeneity regarding imaging features of HEHE. The liver lesions are typically hypoechoic on US, hypodense on CT and usually hypointense on T1-weighted images and hyperintense on T2-weighted images with a target-like

G. Zamboni, S. Gourtsoyianni, *MDCT and MRI of the Liver, Bile Ducts and Pancreas*, A-Z Notes in Radiological Practice and Reporting, DOI 10.1007/978-88-470-5720-3_8,

appearance also reported. A hypointense centre may correspond to calcification, necrosis and haemorrhage. Moderate peripheral enhancement and delayed central enhancement are seen.

Definitive diagnosis of HEHE is established by immunohistochemical evidence of endothelial differentiation.

Haemangioma

Haemangioma is the most common benign liver tumour, comprised of interconnected endothelial-lined vascular channels, enclosed within loose fibroblastic stroma and fed by hepatic artery branches.

At nonenhanced CT haemangiomas appear as hypodense well-defined lesions. After contrast administration, early nodular peripheral enhancement is seen, followed by slow centripetal fill-in. In the delayed phase, the lesion is isodense or slightly hyperdense to the adjacent parenchyma.

At MRI, haemangiomas characteristically present with a very long T2 relaxation and appear hypointense on T1-weighted images. Large haemangiomas are usually heterogeneous, containing various combinations of fibrosis, haemorrhage, thrombosis, hyalinisation and cystic degeneration. Typical imaging findings are early hyperintense peripheral nodular enhancement with complete fill-in on delayed imaging.

When small, haemangiomas usually present with uniform early enhancement. Persistent central hypointensity occurs due to fibrosis, thrombosis or degeneration.

Haemochromatosis

In the primary or genetic form of haemochromatosis, there is excessive absorption of iron in the intestine, which cannot be eliminated by the body and accumulates in various organs, causing irreversible damage. In the secondary form, the excess in iron comes from multiple blood transfusions or blood disorders, such as haemolytic anaemia.

The magnitude of body iron stores distinguishes patients who will benefit from treatment from those merely at risk for the disease. MRI is the most sensitive and accurate method to demonstrate and quantify iron overload by using dedicated T2* GRE imaging with different echo times that allow for precise quantification of iron deposition in μmol /g (T2* relaxometry). Liver signal decrease is proportional to the magnetic susceptibility changes induced by iron. T2 relaxometry is the best method to quantify liver iron concentration using MRI. It is accurate and reproducible at all levels of iron overload and also allows myocardial iron concentration to be measured. However, T2 relaxometry models are not yet standardised nor are widely available. On the other hand, signal intensity ratio (SIR) methods, measuring SIR between the liver and other tissues in which iron is not generally deposited, usually paraspinal muscles, although less accurate with values of liver iron concentration >350 μmol Fe/g, have high specificity at all levels of iron overload, have been standardised, are reproducible and are already widely available.

In haemochromatosis the pancreas and myocardium may also be involved but not the spleen. Pancreatic involvement aids in differentiation between cirrhosis with liver iron overload and haemochromatosis with secondary cirrhosis. Hereditary haemochromatosis is associated with an increased risk of HCC.

Hepatic Abscess

Hepatic abscesses appear as isolated or multiple, focal, cystic, liver lesions presenting with thick enhancing capsule on cross-sectional imaging in a patient that is usually febrile.

Hepatic abscess may be due to biliary tree infection and ascending abdominal infections (appendicitis, diverticulitis, IBD) or secondary to RF or transarterial chemoembolisation with immunosuppressed patients being more prone. Appearances depend on the pathogen, with *Candida* producing multiple small abscesses (<5 mm).

On ultrasound hepatic abscess presents as a hypoechoic to anechoic round mass that might contain septa and debris. Presence of gas is hyperechoic with an acoustic shadow.

At CT, liver abscesses present with peripheral enhancement and central low density. They can occasionally appear solid.

At MRI, they appear heterogeneously hypointense on T1-weighted images and hyperintense on T2-weighted images, with peripheral enhancement. On DWI-MRI abscesses show restricted diffusion on higher b-value images and low ADC values.

Hepatic Adenoma

Hepatic adenoma is a rare benign liver tumour, containing well-differentiated hepatocytes but lacking bile ducts or portal tract. It is seen most commonly in patients with previous history of oestrogen intake (e.g. oral contraception), androgen steroid therapy or underlying metabolic disease. Eighty percent are solitary, when multiple (usually >10 adenomas) the condition is known as hepatic adenomatosis. There is female predominance.

Adenomas are asymptomatic until they present with pain, bleeding and rupture (malignant potential). If size > 3–5 cm, surgery should be considered.

On non-contrast CT, the lesions can appear isodense, hypodense due to the fat component or hyperdense due to haemorrhage.

At MRI, non-haemorrhagic lesions have variable T1 intensity and appear mildly hyperintense on T2-weighted images.

Chemical shift imaging characteristically shows a drop of signal in the out-of-phase images.

After contrast administration, adenomas demonstrate moderate arterial enhancement and washout in the portal venous phase.

When using hepatocyte-specific MRI contrast agents, adenoma typically appears hypointense in the hepatocellular phase.

Hepatocellular adenomas show less enhancement than FNH and typically lack the central scar.

Hepatic Cyst

Hepatic cysts are incidental focal liver lesions picked up on ultrasound or cross-sectional imaging. They can be isolated or multiple, usually in autosomal dominant polycystic disease.

They appear anechoic with marked acoustic enhancement on ultrasound, present low, fluid attenuation (0–10 HU) on CT and are hypointense on T1 and hyperintense on T2-weighted images.

Cysts are surrounded by a thin nonenhancing capsule and are sharply demarcated from the surrounding liver parenchyma. When haemorrhagic, they may be hyperdense on CT and hyperintense on T1-w images. When infected, they present with an enhancing thickened wall.

Hepatitis

Chronic hepatitis does not alter the macroscopic architecture of the liver.

Three types of liver parenchyma enhancement pattern have been described based on gadolinium-enhanced dynamic MRI examination in patients with chronic hepatitis: homogeneous, linear and patchy. Presence of early patchy enhancement indicates either concurrent or recent hepatocellular damage, whereas the presence of late linear enhancement indicates the presence of fibrosis, with a high degree of correlation with histopathologic findings.

Advanced cirrhosis resulting from chronic hepatitis presents with typical morphologic changes in the liver parenchyma and contour.

Hepatocellular Carcinoma

Hepatocellular carcinoma (HCC) is the predominant primary liver cancer worldwide.

Cirrhotic Patient

On T1-w images, HCC usually appears as a hypointense nodule, due to hypercellularity.

However, small well-differentiated HCCs may present as T1-w hyperintense or isointense, due to intracellular presence of glycogen and fat, as in the case of high-grade dysplastic nodule, or due to haemorrhagic changes, although this is quite rarely encountered in larger tumours.

On T2-w, mild signal hyperintensity is shown, while small and well-differentiated HCCs may appear isointense. T2-w signal intensity of the nodule is significantly associated with nodular blood supply: signal increases as portal venous supply decreases.

A capsule may be present. Typical signal behaviour of HCC at post-contrast dynamic study is that of early arterial enhancement (rapid wash in) followed by rapid washout during portal venous phase and late phases. In small well-differentiated HCCs, avid hypervascularity may not be seen.

Non-cirrhotic Patient

HCC in non-cirrhotic patients is more likely to present as a large, solitary or dominant mass that is well defined and has a capsule that is prone to spontaneous rupture and haemoperitoneum. At MRI the lesion shares the same signal characteristics as the one in the cirrhotic patient; however necrotic and haemorrhagic phenomena within the lesion are more frequently encountered due to the size of the lesion at diagnosis.

Hepatospecific MRI Contrast Agents

Liver-specific contrast agents are hepatocyte selective or target specifically Kupffer cells of the reticuloendothelial system in the liver.

Gadobenate dimeglumine (MultiHance®, Gd-BOPTA; Bracco Diagnostics), gadoxetic acid (Primovist®, Gd-EOB-DTPA; Schering AG) and mangafodipir trisodium (Teslascan®, Mn-DPDP; GE Healthcare) are hepatocyte-specific contrast agents that are taken up by hepatocytes and act mainly by shortening T1 relaxation time and enhancing T1-weighted image signal intensity during delayed imaging. These allow for dynamic imaging, like standard extracellular contrast agents, as well as provide a delayed hepatobiliary phase that allows for better characterisation and detection of focal liver lesions.

Clinical indications are characterisation of FNH and adenomas, as these are hyperintense in the hepatobiliary phase, increasing diagnostic confidence. Excretion through biliary ductal system allows for functional information such as depiction of complications from surgical procedures involving the biliary system, while their use has shown an increase in sensitivity for the detection of HCCs < 1 cm.

Hereditary Haemorrhagic Telangiectasia

Hereditary haemorrhagic telangiectasia is an autosomal dominant multiorgan disorder that causes production of fragile telangiectatic vessels and arteriovenous malformations, with a hyperdynamic circulation from shunting.

Patients present with dilated hepatic and portal veins with prominent intrahepatic vascular shunts that may present as confluent vascular masses.

In the arterial phase, heterogeneous enhancement with numerous areas of transient hepatic enhancement difference indicative of arterioportal shunt is seen. Telangiectasias appear as small peripheral perfusion abnormalities during the arterial phase.

Hereditary Pancreatitis

Hereditary pancreatitis is a rare disease, which accounts for 10–15 % of all cases of chronic pancreatitis.

It is an autosomal dominant condition with 80 % penetrance. Several different mutations have been recognised: mutations in the cationic trypsinogen gene (PRSS1), in the cystic fibrosis transmembrane conductance regulator gene (CFTR) or in the serine protease inhibitor Kazal type 1 gene (SPINK1).

These patients undergo recurrent attacks of acute pancreatitis and have a significantly higher risk (53×) of developing pancreatic cancer compared to other forms of chronic pancreatitis.

Hereditary pancreatitis is characterised by the presence of calcifications. The onset of these calcifications is influenced by alcohol, even in small amounts, and cigarette smoke. Pancreatic calcifications are more frequent at least 2 years after the onset of symptoms. These stones are larger than those observed in other forms of chronic pancreatitis and have the typical "bull's-eye" appearance, i.e. with peripheral dense margins and a central lucent core (Fig. 1). This pattern was first described in 1981 by Rohrmann, who observed it on plain films of the abdomen in three patients affected by hereditary chronic pancreatitis. Hoshina confirmed the same finding on ERCP, describing the same "bull's-eye" pattern ductal calculi in three generations of patients with hereditary chronic pancreatitis.

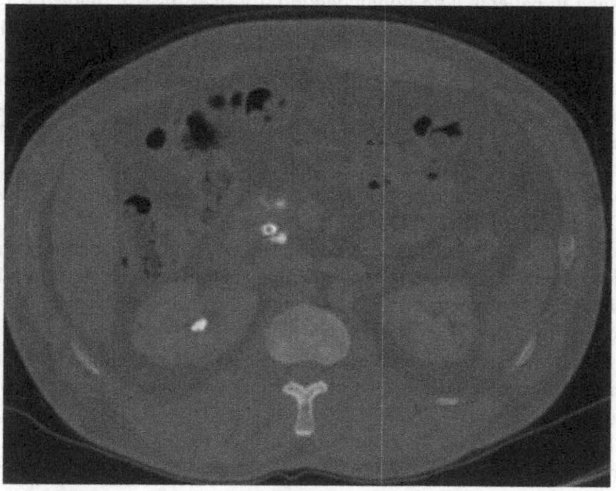

Fig. 1 Hereditary pancreatitis. Multiple calculi are seen in the head of the pancreas, with a central hypodense core and a hyperdense rim, giving the pathognomonic "bull's-eye" appearance

Suggested Reading

Ahn SS, Kim MJ, Lim JS et al (2010) Added value of gadoxetic acid-enhanced hepatobiliary phase MR imaging in the diagnosis of hepatocellular carcinoma. Radiology 255(2):459–66

Alústiza Echeverría JM, Castiella A et al (2012) Quantification of iron concentration in the liver by MRI. Insights Imaging 3(2):173–80

Campos JT, Sirlin CB, Choi JY (2012) Focal hepatic lesions in Gd-EOB-DTPA enhanced MRI: the atlas. Insights Imaging. 3(5):451–74

Caseiro-Alves F, Brito J, Araujo AE et al (2007) Liver haemangioma: common and uncommon findings and how to improve the differential diagnosis. Eur Radiol 17(6):1544–54

Graziani R, Manfredi R, Cicero C et al (2010) Role of multislice computed tomography in the diagnosis of gene-mutation-associated pancreatitis (GMAP). Radiol Med. 115(6):875–88.

Gupta RT, Brady CM, Lotz J et al (2010) Dynamic MR imaging of the biliary system using hepatocyte-specific contrast agents. AJR Am J Roentgenol 195(2):405–13

Iannaccone R, Piacentini F, Murakami T et al (2007) Hepatocellular carcinoma in patients with nonalcoholic fatty liver disease: helical CT and MR imaging findings with clinical-pathologic comparison. Radiology. 243(2):422–30

Paolantonio P, Laghi A, Vanzulli A, et al (2013) MRI of Hepatic Epithelioid Hemangioendothelioma (HEH). J Magn Reson Imaging 2013 Nov 13 (epub ahead of print)

Perez-Johnston R, Sainani NI, Sahani DV (2012) Imaging of chronic pancreatitis (including groove and autoimmune pancreatitis). Radiol Clin North Am 50(3):447–66

Semelka RC, Chung JJ, Hussain SM et al (2001) Chronic hepatitis: correlation of early patchy and late linear enhancement patterns on gadolinium-enhanced MR images with histopathology initial experience. J Magn Reson Imaging 13(3):385–91

Shinmura R, Matsui O, Kobayashi S et al. (2005) Cirrhotic nodules: association between MR imaging signal intensity and intranodular blood supply. Radiology 237(2):512–9.

Van Beers B, Roche A, Mathieu D et al (1992) Epithelioid hemangioendothelioma of the liver: MR and CT findings. J Comput Assist Tomogr 16(3):420–4.

I

In-Phase and Out-of-Phase Imaging

It is also referred to as chemical shift imaging. Varying the TE of T1-w GRE sequence in-phase (fat and water protons in phase) and out-of-phase (net cancellation of signal: drop of signal intensity in fat-containing areas/lesions) images may be obtained which provide information on parenchymal and lesion fat content (Fig. 1). Opposed-phase images have a shorter TE, normal liver is brighter, and fat-containing areas/lesions demonstrate decrease in signal intensity.

Inflammatory Pseudotumours (Liver)

Liver inflammatory pseudotumours are rare, benign liver lesions containing fibroblasts, collagen and inflammatory cells that usually present as large infiltrative tumours on imaging with abnormal liver function tests.

G. Zamboni, S. Gourtsoyianni, *MDCT and MRI of the Liver, Bile Ducts and Pancreas*, A-Z Notes in Radiological Practice and Reporting, DOI 10.1007/978-88-470-5720-3_9,

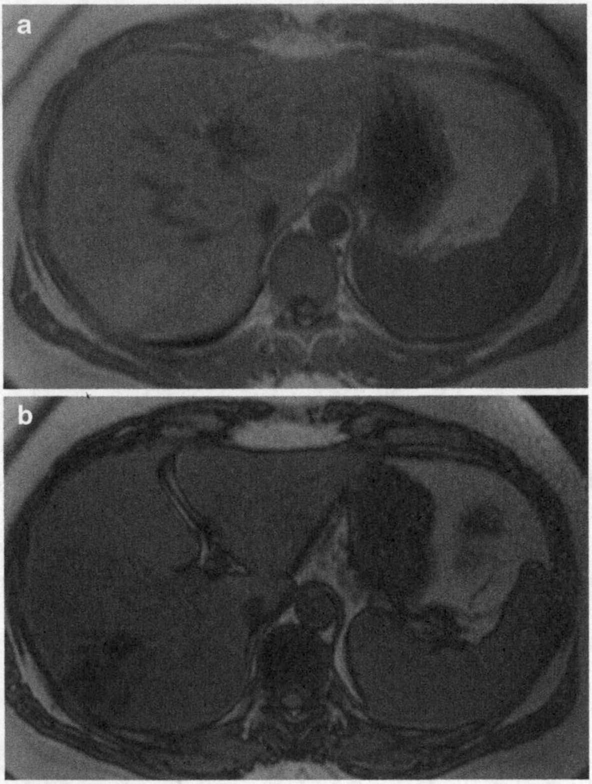

Fig. 1 In phase and out of phase: T1-w GE in-phase (**a**) and out-of-phase (**b**) imaging is very useful for characterisation of focal hepatic steatosis by demonstrating signal drop

Two different patterns have been described: ill-defined, numerous, T2-w hyperintense, active liver lesions and T2-w hypointense lesions, holding a capsule, during nonactive phase.

Biopsy may be required to differentiate from cholangiocarcinoma. They regress spontaneously or after treatment with corticosteroids.

IPMN

Intraductal papillary mucinous neoplasm, the most common cystic tumour of the pancreas, is a mucin-producing tumour originating from the epithelium of the main pancreatic duct (main duct type), its side branches (side-branch type) or both (combined type).

IPMNs are typically diagnosed in males, mainly in the seventh decade.

Main-duct IPMNs are always to be considered malignant lesions and appear as an irregularly dilated duct, involving the MPD entirely or segmentally, with content that is hyperintense on T2-weighted images and hypointense on T1-weighted images (Fig. 2).

Branch-duct IPMNs should be considered malignant when enhancing nodules are visualised or when the tumour size exceeds 3 cm. Branch-duct IPMNs appear as round or oval accumulations of mucin, most common in the head or uncinated process, without a well-defined wall, hyperintense to the pancreatic parenchyma on T2-weighted images and hypointense on T1-weighted images.

The most important imaging clue for the diagnosis of branch-duct IPMN is the visualisation of the communication with the main pancreatic duct, which is highly specific for this diagnosis; MRCP can be very helpful in identifying this communication.

Combined-type IPMNs will show a combination of main ductal dilatation and dilatation of side branches.

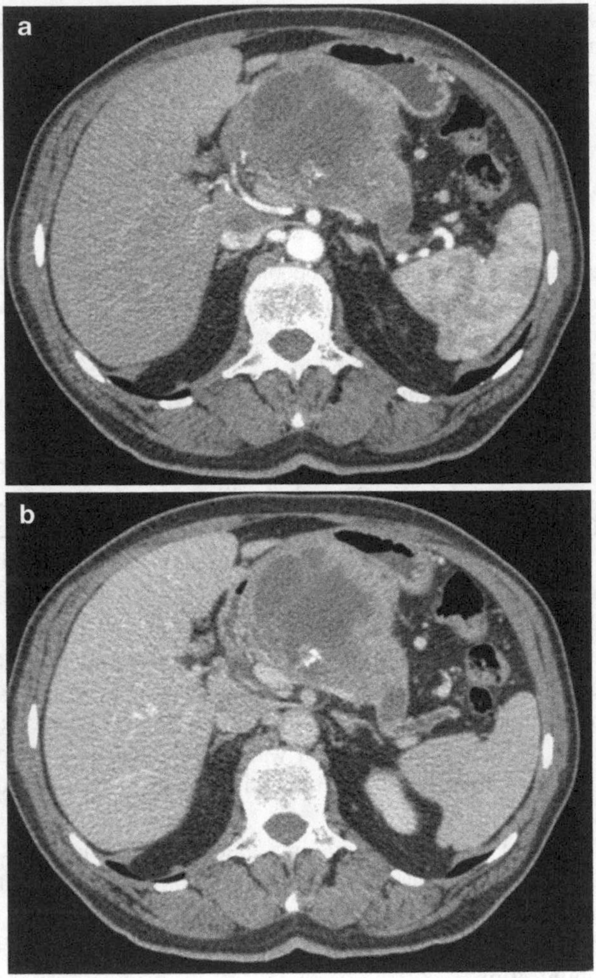

Fig. 2 Main-duct IPMN. Axial arterial (**a**) and portal venous (**b**) CT images show a large cystic dilatation of the main pancreatic duct in the body–tail, with enhancing mural nodules and coarse calcifications

After gadolinium administration, the enhancement of eventual intraluminal nodules or thickened wall can be visualised. Gadolinium administration can aid in the differential diagnosis between solid mural nodules and mucin globules.

Suggested Reading

Kim KW, Park SH, Pyo J et al (2014) Imaging features to distinguish malignant and benign branch-duct type intraductal papillary mucinous neoplasms of the pancreas: a meta-analysis. Ann Surg. 259(1):72–81

Manfredi R, Graziani R, Motton M et al (2009) Main pancreatic duct intraductal papillary mucinous neoplasms: accuracy of MR imaging in differentiation between benign and malignant tumors compared with histopathologic analysis. Radiology 253(1):106–15.

Procacci C, Carbognin G, Biasiutti C et al (2001) Intraductal papillary mucinous tumors of the pancreas: spectrum of CT and MR findings with pathologic correlation. Eur Radiol. 11(10):1939–51.

Procacci C, Megibow AJ, Carbognin G et al (1999) Intraductal papillary mucinous tumor of the pancreas: a pictorial essay. Radiographics 19(6): 1447–63.

J

No Lemma

G. Zamboni, S. Gourtsoyianni, *MDCT and MRI of the Liver, Bile Ducts and Pancreas*, A-Z Notes in Radiological Practice and Reporting, DOI 10.1007/978-88-470-5720-3_10,

K

No Lemma

G. Zamboni, S. Gourtsoyianni, *MDCT and MRI of the Liver, Bile Ducts and Pancreas*, A-Z Notes in Radiological Practice and Reporting, DOI 10.1007/978-88-470-5720-3_11,

L

Lymphoma, Liver

Primary lymphoma is very rare. Secondary lymphoma of the liver is encountered in more than 50 % of patients with Hodgkin and non-Hodgkin lymphoma. On MRI focal deposits present with T1-w hypointense and T2-w hyperintense signal intensity. Transient perilesional enhancement has been reported.

Lymphoma, Pancreas

Pancreatic lymphoma is most commonly a B-cell subtype of non-Hodgkin lymphoma and can be classified as either primary or secondary. Primary pancreatic lymphoma is rare, representing less than 0.5 % of pancreatic tumours. Secondary lymphoma of the pancreas can be seen in up to 30 % of patients with widespread non-Hodgkin lymphoma.

G. Zamboni, S. Gourtsoyianni, *MDCT and MRI of the Liver, Bile Ducts and Pancreas*, A-Z Notes in Radiological Practice and Reporting, DOI 10.1007/978-88-470-5720-3_12,

Pancreatic lymphoma typically affects middle-aged patients and immunocompromised patients, with an incidence as high as 5 % in human immunodeficiency virus (HIV) patients. The presentation is often non-specific, without the typical symptoms of lymphoma.

Pancreatic lymphoma can present in a diffuse (16.7 %) or in a focal form (66.7 %). The diffuse form is characterised by organ enlargement, without a well-defined mass, while the focal form occurs most often in the pancreatic head (80 %).

CT shows focal or diffuse enlargement of the organ, with uniform low attenuation and minimal enhancement (Fig. 1). Peripancreatic nodes may be enlarged, and encasement of the peripancreatic vessels may be seen, although vascular invasion is rare.

At MRI, lymphomatous tissue shows low signal intensity on T1-weighted images, while the intensity on T2-weighted images is variable, from low to high. On T2-WI the lesions can appear heterogeneous. After Gd administration, the contrast enhancement is lower than that of the normal pancreas. No information has been reported yet on the use of DWI for pancreatic lymphoma, although its use for total-body imaging of lymphomas is becoming common.

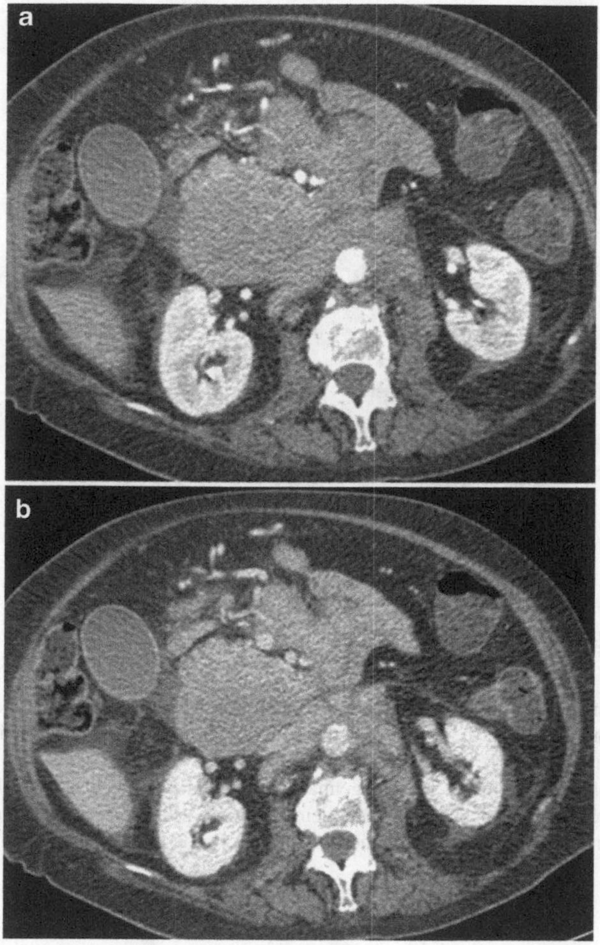

Fig. 1 Axial arterial phase (**a**) and venous phase axial (**b**) and coronal (**c**) images show a large mass in the pancreatic head, with smooth lobulated margins, hypovascular. The choledochus is dilated. Multiple enlarged lymph nodes are appreciated in the retroperitoneum

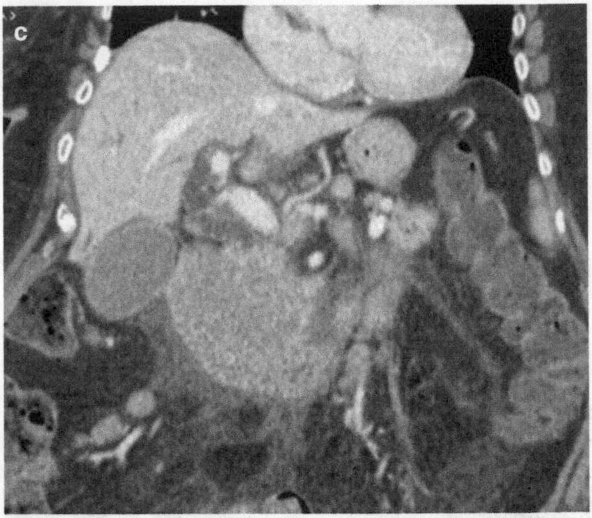

Fig. 1 (continued)

Suggested Reading

Fujinaga Y, Lall C, Patel A et al (2013) MR features of primary and secondary malignant lymphoma of the pancreas: a pictorial review. Insights Imaging 4(3):321–9

Kelekis NL, Semelka RC, Siegelman ES et al (1997) Focal hepatic lymphoma: magnetic resonance demonstration using current techniques including gadolinium enhancement. Magn Reson Imaging 15(6):625–36.

M

MEN

Multiple endocrine neoplasia (MEN) syndromes are a collection of autosomal dominant syndromes characterised by the presence of multiple endocrine tumours.

Multiple endocrine neoplasia (MEN) type I, also known as Wermer syndrome, is characterised by parathyroid hyperplasia, islet cell tumours of the pancreas (most often gastrinomas, followed by glucagonomas) and pituitary adenomas.

MEN type II is associated with medullary thyroid cancer, parathyroid tumours and pheochromocytoma.

Metastases, Liver

Liver is the second most frequent metastatic site, with liver metastases being the most common form of malignant liver disease. The single best examination with lower rate of further imaging for therapy decision in case of liver metastasis detection has been shown to be EOB-DTPA MRI, compared to

G. Zamboni, S. Gourtsoyianni, *MDCT and MRI of the Liver, Bile Ducts and Pancreas*, A-Z Notes in Radiological Practice and Reporting, DOI 10.1007/978-88-470-5720-3_13,

extracellular contrast agent MRI and triple-phase MDCT examination.

Thyroid carcinoma, carcinoid, neuroendocrine tumours, RCC and to a lesser extent pancreas, breast and colon cancer and cancer of unknown primary give hypervascular liver metastases at early dynamic phase, which then demonstrate typical washout on portal venous phase (Fig. 1).

Hypovascular liver metastases encountered predominantly in colon, lung, breast and gastric primaries are hypointense on all phases and may demonstrate perilesional enhancement in the arterial phase due to peritumoral desmoplastic reaction, presence of inflammatory cells and vascular proliferation.

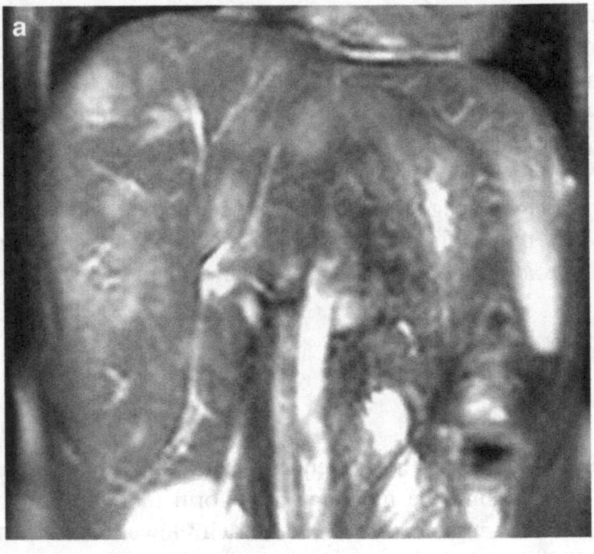

Fig. 1 Liver metastases: multiple T2-w hyperintense liver lesions are noted in both liver lobes (**a**) that present with restricted diffusion (high signal intensity on **b** 800 image **b**, low signal intensity on corresponding ADC map (**c**) and demonstrate enhancement pattern typical for liver metastases (**d**). The patient was found to have a small bowel carcinoid

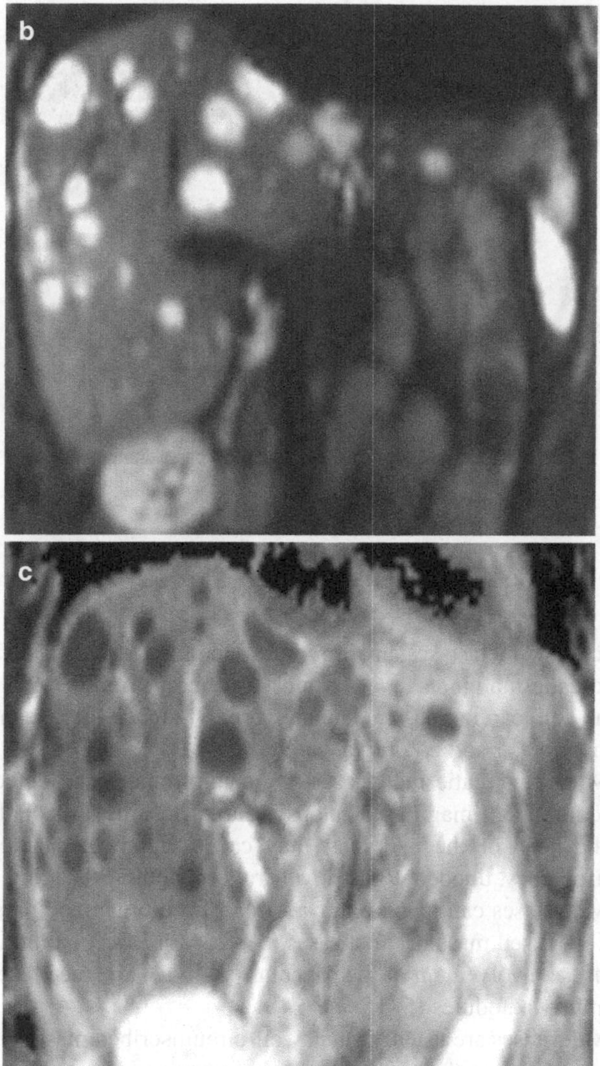

Fig. 1 (continued)

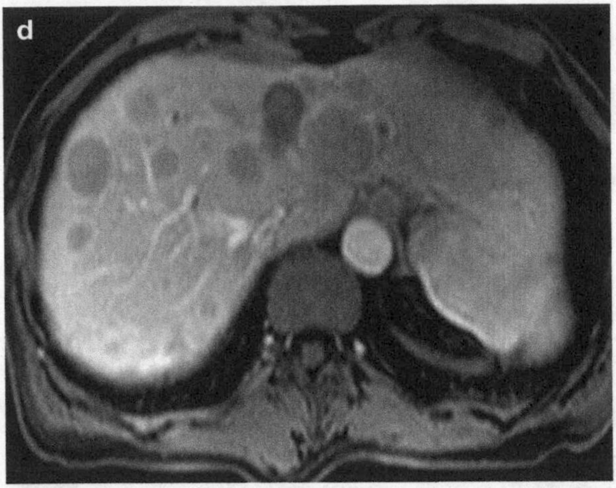

Fig. 1 (continued)

Metastases, Pancreas

Pancreatic metastases are rare and account for 2–5 % of all pancreatic malignancies. The most common primaries include renal cell carcinoma, melanoma, breast cancer, lung cancer, gastric cancer and colorectal carcinoma.

Most pancreatic metastases are asymptomatic and detected incidentally at imaging or autopsy. Larger lesions, especially if in the head of the pancreas, may cause jaundice, pancreatic insufficiency, duodenal/gastric obstruction and GI bleeding.

Metastases can involve any portion of the organ and present as a localised mass in most cases (50–75 %). Less common are a diffuse involvement of the pancreas (5–45 %) and the presence of multiple nodules (5–15 %).

Metastases are usually small well-circumscribed masses, iso- to hypodense to the normal parenchyma on non-contrast scans. Calcifications are rare. Post-contrast enhancement resembles

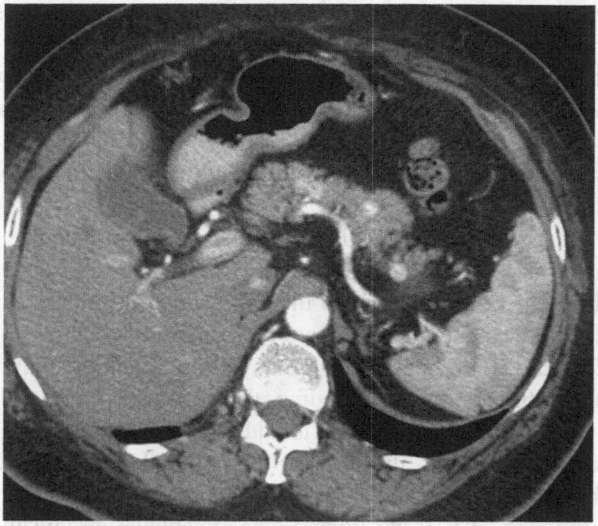

Fig. 2 Pancreatic metastases: arterial phase CT shows multiple small hypervascular pancreatic lesions, consistent with metastases in a patient with history of renal cell carcinoma

that of the primary tumour and is usually homogeneous in smaller lesions and peripheral in larger lesions, presumably due to central necrosis (Fig. 2).

Metastases in the head of the pancreas commonly cause pancreatic ductal obstruction and may be associated with common bile duct obstruction.

Mirizzi Syndrome

The Mirizzi syndrome refers to obstruction of the common hepatic duct caused by an extrinsic compression from an impacted stone in the cystic duct or Hartmann's pouch of the gallbladder. It was initially described by the Argentinian surgeon Pablo Luis Mirizzi in 1948.

It is a functional hepatic syndrome but can often present with biliary duct dilatation and can mimic other hepatobiliary pathology such as cholangiocarcinoma.

Risk factors include a low insertion of the cystic duct into the common bile duct.

Patients may present with recurrent episodes of jaundice and cholangitis. It can be associated with acute cholecystitis. Fistulae can develop between the gallbladder and the common duct, and the stone may pass into the common duct.

Typical CT findings of Mirizzi syndrome include dilatation of the biliary system, including the common hepatic duct, upstream to the level of the gallbladder neck, the presence of an impacted calculus in the neck of the gallbladder, a contracted gallbladder and a normal calibre of the common bile duct downstream to the level of the stone. Signs of acute or chronic cholecystitis or pericholecystitis may also be present.

MRI with MRCP typically shows the impacted stone in the gallbladder neck, causing compression of the common hepatic duct and dilatation of the biliary system upstream to the level of impaction. The gallbladder is contracted, with thickened walls.

Different classifications have been proposed for the different types of Mirizzi syndrome, the most recent being devised by Csendes:

Type I: extrinsic compression of CHD due to a stone in the cystic duct or in the gallbladder infundibulum.

Type II: cholecystobiliary fistula involving less than 1/3 of the circumference of the bile duct wall.

Type III: cholecystobiliary fistula involving up to two-thirds of the bile duct circumference.

Type IV: cholecystobiliary fistula with complete destruction of the bile duct wall, with the gallbladder completely fused to the bile duct forming a single structure with no recognisable dissection planes.

Type V: presence of a cholecystoenteric fistula together with any other type of Mirizzi. Mirizzi type Va includes a cholecystoenteric fistula without gallstone ileus, while Mirizzi type Vb refers to a cholecystoenteric fistula complicated by gallstone ileus.

MRCP

Magnetic resonance cholangiopancreatography is a non-invasive imaging modality of the pancreatico-biliary system which plays an important role in the clinical and diagnostic workup of patients with biliary or pancreatic diseases. Heavily T2-weighted sequences, such as single-shot fast spin echo (SSFSE), half-Fourier single-shot turbo spin echo (HASTE) and rapid acquisition relaxation enhanced (RARE), are utilised, taking advantage of the long T2 relaxation time of static bile and pancreatic duct fluid to create a road map of the biliary and pancreatic duct system.

Main clinical indications are depiction of stones within the biliary tree, as these appear as low signal intensity filling defects within the bright biliary tree, and biliary strictures.

Maximum intensity projection images (MIPs) are created that simulate ERCP images, with only limitation being the visualization of the ampullary region. No intravenous contrast agent is required. Artefacts encountered within the biliary tree are mostly due to presence of gas, clot, metallic clips, motion or pulsation from crossing vessels.

Negative oral contrast agents can be administered (e.g. iron oxide, pineapple juice or blueberry juice) to reduce the signal intensity of overlapping fluid in the stomach and duodenum.

Delayed T1-weighted fat-saturated GRE images obtained in the axial and coronal planes, acquired 10–120 min after hepatobiliary excretion contrast administration, depending on contrast agent used, allow for demonstration of the communication between cystic lesions and bile ducts in congenital biliary diseases, for differential diagnosis between true obstruction and pseudo-obstruction in a dilated biliary system and for demonstrating active extravasation of contrast in suspected bile leaks. The pancreatic ducts are of course not visualised.

Mucinous Cystic Neoplasms

Mucinous cystic neoplasms account for 10 % of all cystic pancreatic lesions and range from benign (mucinous cystadenoma) to borderline to malignant forms. MCN are usually incidental findings, diagnosed in the 4th–5th decade of life and occur almost exclusively in females. The mucin-producing epithelium is surrounded by ovarian-like stroma, which justifies the strong female prevalence and the preferred location in the body or tail of the pancreas, which is located next to the female gonad during the embryologic development.

Eighty percent are unilocular and 20 % multilocular.

At CT, MCN usually appear rounded or ovoid, with smooth margins. When present, calcifications tend to be peripheral. The cyst content can be inhomogeneous, and internal septations may be present (Fig. 3).

At MR, MCN show well-defined margins. The cyst signal intensity depends on the proportion of mucoid and haemorrhagic components. Usually MCN are homogeneously hyperintense on T2-weighted images. After intravenous gadolinium-chelate administration, the walls enhance on delayed T1-weighted images. Enhancing parietal vegetations or septa with papillary projections into the lumen are highly suspicious for malignant transformation. MRCP can be useful in ruling out a communication with the main pancreatic duct.

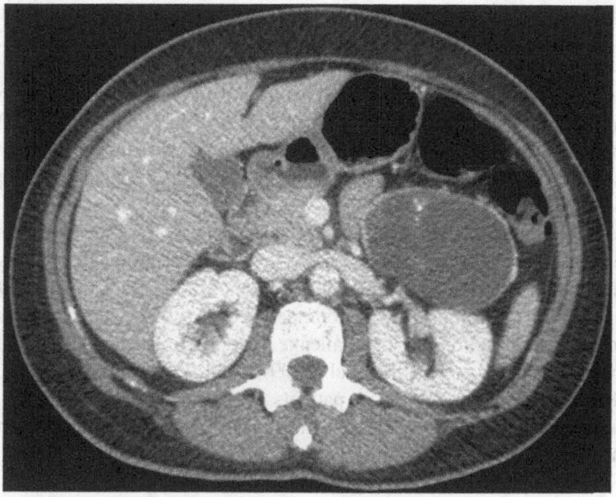

Fig. 3 Mucinous cystic neoplasm. Axial venous phase CT shows a large cystic lesion of the pancreatic tail, with septa that enhance and have calcifications

Features associated with malignancy include age over 55 years, size over 4 cm, associated enhancing mass and eggshell calcifications.

Suggested Reading

Becker CD, Grossholz M, Becker M et al(1997) Choledocholithiasis and bile duct stenosis: diagnostic accuracy of MR cholangiopancreatography. Radiology 205(2):523–30.

Buetow PC, Rao P, Thompson LD (1998) From the Archives of the AFIP. Mucinous cystic neoplasms of the pancreas: radiologic-pathologic correlation. Radiographics 18(2):433–49.

Csendes A, Díaz JC, Burdiles P et al (1989) Mirizzi syndrome and cholecystobiliary fistula: a unifying classification. Br J Surg. 76:1139–1143

Griffin N, Charles-Edwards G, Grant LA (2012) Magnetic resonance cholangiopancreatography: the ABC of MRCP. Insights Imaging. 3(1): 11–21.

Procacci C, Carbognin G, Accordini S et al (2001) CT features of malignant mucinous cystic tumors of the pancreas. Eur Radiol 11(9):1626–30.

Sahni VA, Mortele KJ (2008) Magnetic resonance cholangiopancreatography: current use and future applications. Clin Gastroenterol Hepatol 6(9):967–77

Semelka RC,Hussain SM, Marcos HB, Woosley JT (2000) Perilesional enhancement of hepatic metastases: correlation between MR imaging and histopathologic findings-initial observations. Radiology 215(1):89–94.

Triantopoulou C, Kolliakou E, Karoumpalis I et al (2012) Metastatic disease to the pancreas: an imaging challenge. Insights Imaging 3(2):165–72

Zech CJ, Grazioli L, Jonas E, et al (2009) Health- economic evaluation of three imaging strategies in patients with suspected colorectal liver metastases: Gd-EOB-DTPA-enhanced MRI vs. extracellular contrast media-enhanced MRI and 3-phase MDCT in Germany, Italy and Sweden. Eur Radiol 19 Suppl 3:S753–63.

N

Nodular Regenerative Hyperplasia (NRH)

Benign micronodular transformation of liver parenchyma without fibrosis associated with wide spectrum of systemic diseases and drugs. It is usually clinically asymptomatic and is discovered incidentally during imaging or may present with cholestasis and portal hypertension.

Lobulated liver contour and portal hypertension imaging findings may be present. It may also present with pseudotumoral appearances demonstrating nodules of variable T1-weighted intensity that are T2 weighted hypointense and show variable enhancement. Confirmation with histology is required to differentiate from metastases.

G. Zamboni, S. Gourtsoyianni, *MDCT and MRI of the Liver, Bile Ducts and Pancreas*, A-Z Notes in Radiological Practice and Reporting, DOI 10.1007/978-88-470-5720-3_14,

O

No Lemma

G. Zamboni, S. Gourtsoyianni, *MDCT and MRI of the Liver, Bile Ducts and Pancreas*, A-Z Notes in Radiological Practice and Reporting, DOI 10.1007/978-88-470-5720-3_15,

P

Pancreas Divisum

The most common anatomical variant of the pancreas, it is caused by failure of the ducts of the dorsal and ventral buds to fuse during embryologic development. The prevalence is between 4 and 15 %.

In the most common classic form of pancreas divisum, the small ventral duct (duct of Wirsung) drains via the major papilla and the large dorsal duct (duct of Santorini) drains via the minor papilla (Fig. 1).

Other more rare variants include incomplete pancreas divisum, where a small branch connects the ventral and dorsal pancreas, pancreas divisum with nonpatent major papilla, where the entire pancreatic ductal system drains via the minor papilla, and reversed pancreas divisum, where the small dorsal duct drains through the minor papilla, while the large ventral duct drains through the major papilla.

Most patients with pancreas divisum are asymptomatic; however this abnormality is observed more frequently in patients with chronic abdominal pain and chronic pancreatitis than in the general population.

G. Zamboni, S. Gourtsoyianni, *MDCT and MRI of the Liver, Bile Ducts and Pancreas*, A-Z Notes in Radiological Practice and Reporting, DOI 10.1007/978-88-470-5720-3_16,

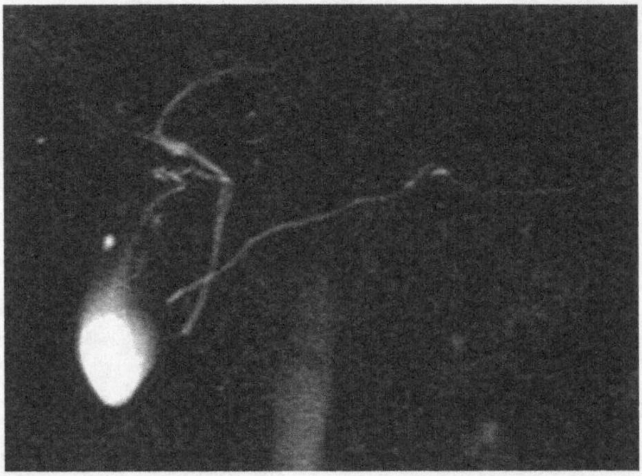

Fig. 1 Pancreas divisum. Coronal thick-slab MRCP image shows the classic form of pancreas divisum, with the large dorsal duct (duct of Santorini) draining via the minor papilla and crossing the choledochus

Pancreatoblastoma

Pancreatoblastoma is the most common pancreatic tumour in the paediatric population.

Pancreatoblastoma usually occurs in the 1st decade of life, with a mean age of 4.5 years at diagnosis. There is slight male predilection (1.3:1 to 2.7:1). It can be associated with Beckwith–Wiedemann syndrome.

Patients most commonly present with an asymptomatic, large abdominal mass; less commonly they present with non-specific complaints. Up to 1/3 of the cases have increased alpha-fetoprotein serum levels.

The tumour occurs most often in the head of the pancreas and tends to be large and solitary. Often at diagnosis the tumour is so large that defining its origin from the pancreas is difficult.

CT usually shows a relatively well-defined and heterogeneous mass. The tumour frequently appears multiloculated with enhancing septa. Small calcifications may be present (punctate, clustered or curvilinear).

At MRI, typically pancreatoblastomas have well-defined margins with low to intermediate signal intensity on T1-weighted images and heterogeneous high signal intensity on T2-weighted images. Necrotic areas appear hypointense on T1 weighted.

Local invasion and dissemination to distant organs may occur. Locally advanced tumours are poorly marginated and invade the surrounding pancreas, the peripancreatic tissues and the adjacent organs. Vascular invasion is rare. Liver and abdominal lymph node metastases are present in 35 % of the patients at diagnosis.

Paraduodenal Pancreatitis

Paraduodenal pancreatitis, previously known as groove pancreatitis, is an uncommon type of focal chronic pancreatitis affecting the potential space between the head of the pancreas, the duodenum and the common bile duct, known as the pancreaticoduodenal groove.

It is a rare disease, seen predominantly in males with a history of alcohol abuse; peak incidence is around 40–50 years.

Two forms of groove pancreatitis have been described: the "pure" form, which affects only the groove, sparing the pancreatic head, and the "segmental" form, which involves the pancreatic head with development of scar tissue within the groove.

CT typically shows hypodense tissue in the pancreaticoduodenal groove, which may demonstrate delayed enhancement. Small cystic lesions may be seen along the medial wall of the duodenum, which is thickened. Common bile duct dilatation may be present.

MR imaging may demonstrate a sheetlike mass in the pancreaticoduodenal groove, usually hypointense to the normal pancreas on T1-weighted images, and with variable intensity on T2-weighted image (hypointense, isointense to slightly hyperintense to the normal pancreas). This tissue, similar to what is observed at CT, may show delayed enhancement after gadolinium administration.

The differential diagnosis is different for the pure and the segmental form.

The pure form enters into differential diagnosis with groove carcinoma, duodenal or periampullary carcinoma, neuroendocrine tumours of the pancreatic groove and acute pancreatitis with inflammatory changes in the groove. A differential diagnosis with pancreatic groove carcinoma is hardly possible on the basis of clinical and imaging features alone, although the presence of cystic lesions within the mass or of a thickened duodenal wall would favour the diagnosis of groove pancreatitis.

The most important differential diagnosis for the segmental form is pancreatic adenocarcinoma: the imaging characteristics of these two diseases may overlap considerably, especially for the scirrhous variant of pancreatic adenocarcinoma, which may demonstrate delayed enhancement similar to groove pancreatitis. Vascular invasion is the most useful sign in differentiating pancreatic adenocarcinoma and groove pancreatitis. MRCP also may reveal a smooth stricture of the distal intrapancreatic portion of the common bile duct in case of groove pancreatitis, while the stricture is abrupt and irregular in case of pancreatic carcinoma.

Peliosis Hepatis

Peliosis hepatis is a rare benign disorder with sinusoidal ectasia and small blood-filled lacunar spaces present in the liver parenchyma. It is usually associated with chronic wasting and infectious diseases (TBC, AIDS), malignancies (HCC, metastases), drugs (steroids, oral contraceptives) or post-transplant immunodeficiency conditions.

Peliotic lesions are usually T2-w hyperintense and may present with haemorrhagic necrosis. Early vessel-like enhancement with persistent enhancement and even isointensity on portal and equilibrium phases may be seen. Centrifugal enhancement, opposite to that of haemangiomas, has been described for peliotic nodules. A branching appearance of vascular component may be observed. After withdrawal of causative agent, peliosis usually regresses.

Portal Vein Thrombosis

Portal vein thrombosis occurs in a variety of clinical settings, the most common of which is liver cirrhosis. Other conditions that may lead to portal vein thrombosis include infectious diseases, tumours, hypercoagulable states, haematologic disorders, surgery and embolism from superior mesenteric or splenic vein thrombosis.

Bland thrombus should be differentiated from tumoral thrombus, which can be present in case of carcinoma: enhancement of the thrombus in the arterial phase is suggestive for its tumoral nature. Neoplastic thrombus also expands the lumen of the portal vein, in contrast to bland thrombus.

Nonenhanced CT in some cases may show focal high attenuation in the portal, superior mesenteric or splenic vein and venous enlargement in case of acute thrombosis. Chronic venous thrombosis can show linear calcifications within the thrombus. Contrast-enhanced CT demonstrates a filling defect that occludes partially or totally the vessel lumen. Rim enhancement of the vessel wall may be seen, presumably due to normal flow in the vasa vasorum.

At MRI, bland thrombus will appear hyperintense on T1-weighted images and hypointense on T2-weighted images, while tumour thrombus is typically hyperintense on T2-WI.

The presence of cavernous transformation of the portal vein, of portosystemic collateral vessels and of arterioportal shunts are indirect signs of portal vein thrombosis.

Portal vein thrombosis is associated with perfusion anomalies of the liver parenchyma, namely, increased arterial inflow and decreased portal vein perfusion. In case of long-standing thrombosis, the increased arterial supply can induce fatty changes in the liver, which appears hypoattenuating.

Primary Biliary Cirrhosis (PBC)

Primary biliary cirrhosis (PBC) is a chronic progressive cholestatic liver disease, presumably autoimmune, that leads to progressive cholestasis and often end-stage liver disease.

Primary biliary cirrhosis is the cause of 1–2 % of deaths from cirrhosis and the third most common indication for liver transplantation in adults. PBC affects most commonly women, between the fourth and sixth decades of life.

The most commonly reported symptoms are fatigue, pruritus and right upper quadrant discomfort, accompanied by laboratory test evidence of cholestasis.

The hallmark of PBC is the presence of serum antimitochondrial antibodies (AMAs), which are present in 90–95 % of patients and have 98 % specificity.

Imaging should first exclude biliary obstruction.

The periportal halo sign has been described as specific for this form of cirrhosis: the presence of conspicuous hypointense abnormalities centred around the portal venous branches on T1- and T2-weighted MR images. The criteria for a positive MRI periportal halo sign include a rounded lesion centred on a portal venous branch (5 mm–1 cm in size) and numerous lesions involving all hepatic segments, with low signal intensity on T1- and T2-weighted images and without mass effect. These criteria allow a differential diagnosis with regenerative nodules, which are usually of various sizes and signal intensity, may exert mass effect and are not centred on portal venous branches. Lymphadenopathy is seen in most patients, especially in the gastrohepatic ligament and porta hepatis.

Other non-specific findings include nodular appearance of the liver, periportal hyperintensity, segmental hypertrophy, varices, splenomegaly and ascites.

DWI has been suggested to be useful in assessing liver fibrosis distribution and for disease staging in cases where liver biopsy is not adequate

Primary Sclerosing Cholangitis

It is a chronic, non-infectious inflammatory disorder of the bile ducts. Smaller biliary radicles are obliterated, and larger biliary radicals develop progressive, irregular strictures leading to cirrhosis, portal hypertension and liver failure. A strong association with inflammatory bowel disease has been reported. Liver biopsy is recommended for staging of PSC. Imaging findings on MRCP are multifocal intra- and extrahepatic bile duct strictures with intervening normal or dilated segments, the so-called *pruned and beaded appearance*.

Dilatation and good visualisation of peripheral ducts on MRCP are considered abnormal due to multiple strictures. MRCP can diagnose PSC but has difficulties in identifying early PSC and in cirrhosis, as well as in the differentiation from cholangiocarcinoma. A positive MRCP would negate a diagnostic ERCP study; however a negative MRCP would not obviate the need for ERCP.

Pseudocyst

Pancreatic pseudocysts are the most common cystic lesions of the pancreas.

They are frequently observed on imaging follow-up of acute pancreatitis and may be symptomatic or may remain asymptomatic for some time. If symptomatic, pseudocysts may cause mass effect (biliary obstruction, gastric outlet obstruction) or may become superinfected.

Pseudocysts are the consequence of a disruption of the pancreatic ductal system, with resulting leakage and accumulation of pancreatic juice. This fluid induces a severe inflammatory reaction, resulting in encapsulation of the cyst with fibrous tissue. This usually happens at least 4 weeks after the onset of the pancreatitis. In approximately half of the cases, the cyst communicates with the pancreatic duct. Pseudocysts are round or oval collections with a fluid content and a relatively thick wall. They can be single or multiple and are most commonly located in the pancreatic area, but they can be found anywhere from the abdomen and pelvis to the mediastinum. The differential diagnosis between an infected and a non-infected pseudocyst is not reliable at imaging.

At CT, pseudocysts appear as rounded masses with fluid density and a uniformly thick wall, with some post-contrast enhancement.

At MRI pseudocysts appear hypointense on T1-WI and hyperintense on T2-WI; dependent debris may be present.

After Gd administration, the cyst wall demonstrates mild early enhancement, which progressively becomes more intense.

Pancreatic pseudocysts enter into differential diagnosis with cystic lesions of the pancreas and with peripancreatic collections of acute pancreatitis (which appear before 4 weeks and are not round but take on the contours of the space in which they are located).

Suggested Reading

Chung EM, Travis MD, Conran RM (2006) Pancreatic tumors in children: radiologic-pathologic correlation. Radiographics 26(4):1211–38

Gallego C, Velasco M, Marcuello P et al (2002) Congenital and acquired anomalies of the portal venous system. Radiographics 22(1):141–59.

Kim YH, Saini S, Sahani D et al (2005) Imaging diagnosis of cystic pancreatic lesions: pseudocyst versus nonpseudocyst. Radiographics 25(3):671–85.

Kovač JD, Ješić R, Stanisavljević D et al (2012) Integrative role of MRI in the evaluation of primary biliary cirrhosis. Eur Radiol. 22(3):688–94

Macari M, Finn ME, Bennett GL et al (2009) Differentiating pancreatic cystic neoplasms from pancreatic pseudocysts at MR imaging: value of perceived internal debris. Radiology 251(1):77–84

Sandrasegaran K, Tahir B, Nutakki K et al (2013) Usefulness of conventional MRI sequences and diffusion-weighted imaging in differentiating malignant from benign portal vein thrombus in cirrhotic patients. AJR Am J Roentgenol 201(6):1211–9

Shet NS, Cole BL, Iyer RS (2014) Imaging of pediatric pancreatic neoplasms with radiologic-histopathologic correlation. AJR Am J Roentgenol. 202(6):1337–48.

Triantopoulou C, Dervenis C, Giannakou N et al (2009) Groove pancreatitis: a diagnostic challenge. Eur Radiol. 19(7):1736–43.

Weber C, Kuhlencordt R, Grotelueschen R et al (2008) Magnetic resonance cholangiopancreatography in the diagnosis of primary sclerosing cholangitis. Endoscopy 40(9):739–45

Wenzel JS, Donohoe A, Ford KL 3rd et al (2001) Primary biliary cirrhosis: MR imaging findings and description of MR imaging periportal halo sign. AJR Am J Roentgenol 176(4):885–9

Q

No Lemma

G. Zamboni, S. Gourtsoyianni, *MDCT and MRI of the Liver, Bile Ducts and Pancreas*, A-Z Notes in Radiological Practice and Reporting, DOI 10.1007/978-88-470-5720-3_17,

R

No Lemma

G. Zamboni, S. Gourtsoyianni, *MDCT and MRI of the Liver, Bile Ducts and Pancreas*, A-Z Notes in Radiological Practice and Reporting, DOI 10.1007/978-88-470-5720-3_18,

S

Secretin MRCP

Secretin is an endogenous hormone normally produced by the duodenum and secreted in response to increased intraluminal acidity, which stimulates the exocrine secretion of the pancreas.

Synthetic human secretin can be administered during MRCP at the dose of 1 ml/10 kg of body weight or 0.2 μg/kg of body weight to induce secretion of bicarbonate-rich fluid from pancreatic ductal cells and a transient increase in the tone of the sphincter of Oddi, resulting in improved visualisation of the pancreatic ductal system.

After intravenous injection, the authors scan patients with a coronal single-shot turbo SE sequence, repeated every 30 s for 10 min. After this interval, a respiratory synchronised 3D turbo SE sequence can be acquired.

The effect of secretin starts immediately and peaks 3–5 min after the injection, when the calibre of the main pancreatic duct is increased by 1 mm or more compared to baseline. After 10 min the calibre of the main pancreatic duct should return to

G. Zamboni, S. Gourtsoyianni, *MDCT and MRI of the Liver, Bile Ducts and Pancreas*, A-Z Notes in Radiological Practice and Reporting, DOI 10.1007/978-88-470-5720-3_19,

baseline; a persistent dilatation of >3 mm is considered abnormal.

Common indications for the use of secretin MRCP include the detection and characterisation of pancreatic ductal anomalies and strictures, characterisation of any communication between the pancreatic duct and cystic lesions, evaluation of the integrity of the pancreatic duct and assessment of pancreatic function and sphincter of Oddi dysfunction.

Serous Cystic Adenoma

Serous cystic adenoma (SCA) is a cystic tumour composed of cysts of different size, containing a fluid with glycogen and various degrees of proteins but no mucin. Based on their morphology, they are classified as having a polycystic (70 % of cases), honeycomb (20 %) or oligocystic pattern (<10 %). SCAs are usually asymptomatic until they become large enough to cause duodenal or common bile duct obstruction; only in these cases surgery should be suggested. At MR imaging, a macrocystic pattern and a size >3 cm at the time of diagnoses can be predictive of lesion enlargement.

Microcystic Serous Cystadenoma

Serous microcystic cystadenoma is a benign pancreatic tumour occurring most commonly in females over 70 years ("the grandmother lesion"). The most common location is the pancreatic head or neck, but they have been described in all locations. SCA is usually an incidental finding at imaging, although larger lesions can cause nausea or abdominal pain. Microcystic serous cystadenoma is composed of multiple small cysts (usually >6) of varying sizes but always less than 2 cm of diameter with the larger cysts located peripherally, separated by thin septa. SCA typically has lobulated margins and does not have a capsule. Punctate or coarse calcifications can be present in more or less 20 % of the cases, usually in lesions larger than 5 cm. At MR imaging these lesions have a typical appearance; therefore further investigations and fine-needle aspiration are usually not required.

CT typically demonstrates a multicystic, lobulated mass in the pancreatic head region. A characteristic enhancing central scar may be present, which can show associated stellate calcifications.

At MRI, the cyst content is hyperintense on T2-weighted images and usually hypointense on T1-weighted images. Sometimes hyperintense areas on T1-WI can be present, due to previous intracystic haemorrhage. Fibrotic components are hypointense on T1-WI. Calcifications are hypointense both on T1- and T2-weighted images. The multiple thin septa radiating from the central scar show strong enhancement after gadolinium administration resulting in the so-called honeycomb-like pattern, with persistent enhancement of the central scar on more delayed scans (Fig. 1). The arteries supplying the tumour are frequently enlarged. On DWI SCAs do not show a significant restriction in diffusion.

Macrocystic Serous Cystadenoma

Macrocystic serous cystadenoma is a rare variant of SCA, occurring usually in female patients over 50 years. They are always benign and are characterised by the presence of unilocular or bilocular cysts greater than 2 cm in size with no central scar. On T2-weighted MR imaging, the lesion appears homogeneously hyperintense without mural nodules, papillary projections or calcifications. At MR imaging, no enhancement

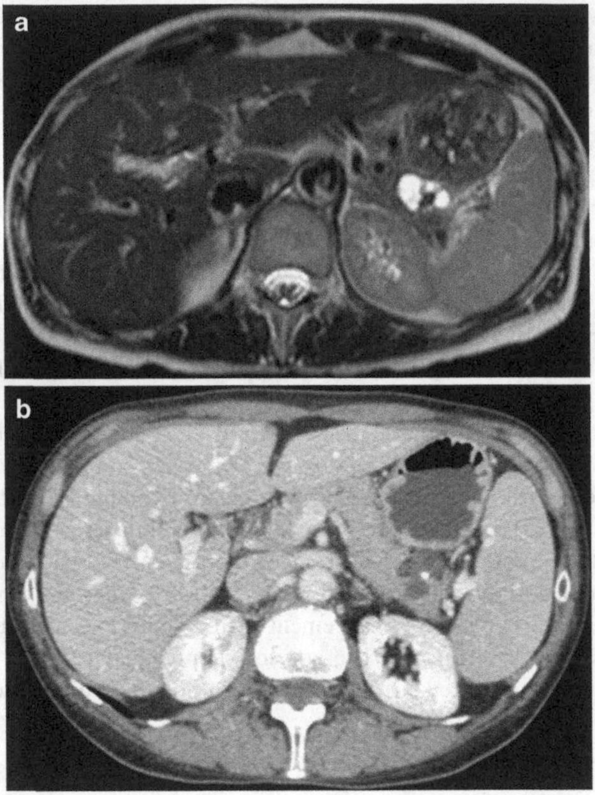

Fig. 1 Serous cystic adenoma. Axial T2-weighted image (**a**) shows a multiloculated cystic lesion in the tail of the pancreas, with hyperintense fluid content and multiple thin radiating septa. A central hypointense area with blooming artefact is observed, consistent with calcification. Venous phase CT (**b**) shows the thin radiating septa, without significant enhancement, and better delineates the calcification

is seen after gadolinium-chelate administration. The presence of large cystic spaces may enter into differential diagnosis with mucinous cystic neoplasms.

Solid Pseudopapillary Neoplasm

Solid pseudopapillary neoplasm (SPN) is an uncommon neoplasm that occurs mainly in women (85–90 %) in the second to fourth decades of life. SPN has been reported also in men, but usually at an older age. The reason underlying this female predominance is still unclear, and no hormone receptors have been found despite sophisticated analyses.

At CT, SPN typically presents as a large well-encapsulated mass, with varying solid and cystic components caused by haemorrhagic degeneration; the entire spectrum from completely solid to almost completely cystic may be encountered and observed. Cystic areas are usually located centrally, while solid areas are located in the periphery of the tumour. Small tumours (<3 cm) most commonly appear as purely solid masses with well-defined margins. Calcifications and enhancing solid areas may be present in the periphery of the mass. On baseline scans SPNs are hypodense; in the pancreatic phase, they enhance less than the normal pancreatic parenchyma, and they enhance gradually in the hepatic venous phase. The presence of a focal discontinuity of the capsule, a large tumour size (>6 cm) and a pancreatic tail location may suggest malignancy, while tumours with amorphous or scattered calcifications and tumours that are mostly solid may be more likely benign.

MRI can be more helpful in the diagnosis, especially in lesions with prevalent cystic components. MRI typically shows a well-defined lesion with a combination of high- and low-signal-intensity areas on T1- and T2-weighted images (Fig. 2). Tumours that are predominantly solid appear mildly hyperintense on T2-weighted images, while those that are mostly cystic appear markedly hyperintense. The identification of blood products can be very helpful and aid in the diagnosis of SPN: areas that are hyperintense on T1-weighted images and homogeneously or inhomogeneously hypointense on T2-weighted

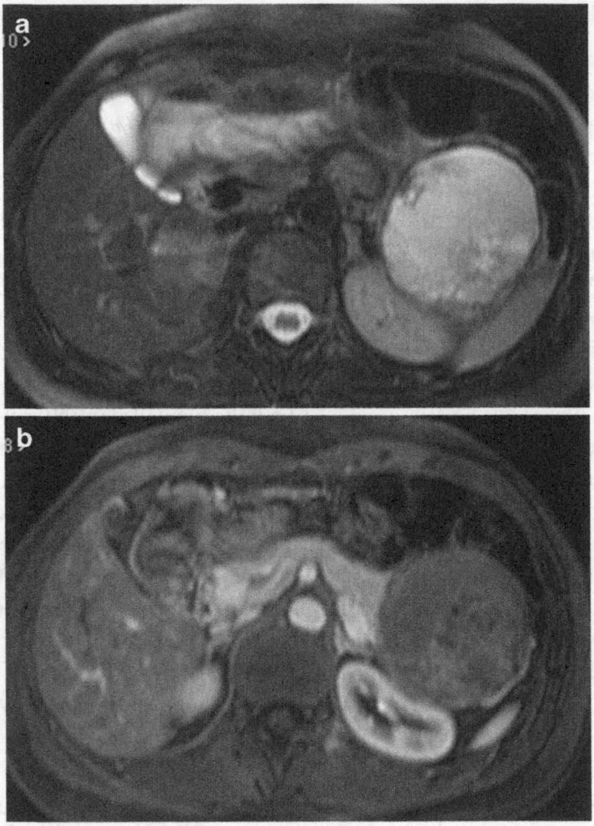

Fig. 2 SPN. Axial T2-weighted image (**a**) shows a large well-defined cystic lesion in the tail of the pancreas, with hyperintense fluid content with some hypointense areas in the dorsal portion. Arterial phase T1-w image after Gd administration shows enhancing papillae within the lesion, consistent with SPN (**b**)

images can be suggestive of blood products. The absence of hyperintensity on T1-weighted images, however, should not exclude the diagnosis. Fluid–fluid levels may be occasionally present. SPNs usually show a fibrous capsule of variable thickness, depicted as a rim of low signal intensity both on T1- and T2-weighted images. After Gd administration, SPNs show early, peripheral and heterogeneous enhancement in the arterial phase with progressive heterogeneous fill-in of the lesion in the portal venous and equilibrium phases. The enhancement is usually inferior to that of the normal parenchyma. In most of the cases, the tumour capsule shows early and more intense enhancement compared with the tumour.

Suggested Reading

Choi JY, Kim MJ, Lee JY et al. (2009) Typical and atypical manifestations of serous cystadenoma of the pancreas: imaging findings with pathologic correlation. Am J Roentgenol 193:136–142

Malleo G, Bassi C, Rossini R et al. (2012) Growth pattern of serous cystic neoplasms of the pancreas: observational study with long-term magnetic resonance surveillance and recommendations for treatment. Gut 61:746–751,

Manfredi R, Bonatti M, D'Onofrio M, et al. (2013) Incidentally discovered benign pancreatic cystic neoplasms not communicating with the ductal system: MR/MRCP imaging appearance and evolution. Radiol Med 118:163–180

Tirkes T, Sandrasegaran K, Sanyal R et al (2013) Secretin-enhanced MR cholangiopancreatography: spectrum of findings. Radiographics 33(7): 1889–906

Zamboni GA, Ambrosetti MC, Pecori S et al (2014) Solid Pseudopapillary Neoplasms. In: D'Onofrio, Capelli, Pederzoli (Eds) Imaging and Pathology of Pancreatic Neoplasms. Springer

T

Teardrop Superior Mesenteric Vein Sign

The teardrop superior mesenteric vein sign is one of the important signs of unresectability of adenocarcinoma of the pancreatic head.

The sign refers to the tethered, teardrop appearance of the SMV when encased by pancreatic head carcinoma, which renders the tumour unresectable.

The sign is highly specific (98 %) for unresectability, with a positive predictive value of 95 %.

Transient Hepatic Attenuation Difference (THAD)

Transient hepatic attenuation difference (THAD) stands for a perfusional liver parenchymal change detected only on the arterial phase of a bolus-enhanced dynamic CT examination that returns to normal on portal venous phase.

G. Zamboni, S. Gourtsoyianni, *MDCT and MRI of the Liver, Bile Ducts and Pancreas*, A-Z Notes in Radiological Practice and Reporting, DOI 10.1007/978-88-470-5720-3_20,

It may involve the entire lobe (lobar), may be segmental or subsegmental or may present within a subcapsular liver location. It may accompany malignant lesions, representing steal syndrome in hypervascular tumours, as well as be associated to non-tumor vascular reasons such as arterioportal shunts and compression of hepatic artery, portal vein or hepatic vein, or accompany benign liver lesions such as haemangioma, FNH, pyogenic abscess and focal eosinophilic necrosis.

Imaging characteristics of benign THAD are those of a wedge-shape, straight line margin focal area with normal vessels crossing through identified only on arterial phase.

Suggested Reading

Hough TJ, Raptopoulos V, Siewert B et al. (1999) Teardrop superior mesenteric vein: CT sign for unresectable carcinoma of the pancreas. AJR Am J Roentgenol. 173(6):1509–12.

Kim HJ, Kim AY, Kim TK et al (2005) Transient hepatic attenuation differences in focal hepatic lesions: dynamic CT features. AJR Am J Roentgenol. 184(1):83–90.

U

No Lemma

G. Zamboni, S. Gourtsoyianni, *MDCT and MRI of the Liver, Bile Ducts and Pancreas*, A-Z Notes in Radiological Practice and Reporting, DOI 10.1007/978-88-470-5720-3_21,

V

von Hippel–Lindau Disease

von Hippel–Lindau (VHL) disease is a hereditary phakomatosis, a rare autosomal dominant neurocutaneous dysplasia complex with 80–100 % penetrance and variable delayed expressivity. It is characterised by visceral cysts and benign tumours in multiple organ systems, with potential for malignant change. Sex distribution is equal, and 20 % of cases are familial.

The clinical hallmarks of von Hippel–Lindau disease are the development of retinal and central nervous system haemangioblastomas, pheochromocytomas and multiple cysts in the pancreas and kidneys and an increased risk for malignant transformation of renal cysts into carcinoma.

The pancreas is involved in up to 77 %. Pancreatic lesions may be the only abdominal manifestation and may precede any other manifestation by several years. The most common lesions are simple pancreatic cysts (91 %), serous cystadenomas (12 %) and neuroendocrine tumours (7–12 %). Pancreatic cysts are extremely rare in the general population: the finding of a single

G. Zamboni, S. Gourtsoyianni, *MDCT and MRI of the Liver, Bile Ducts and Pancreas*, A-Z Notes in Radiological Practice and Reporting, DOI 10.1007/978-88-470-5720-3_22,

cyst while screening subjects with a family history of VHL makes it highly likely that the person is affected by VHL disease.

Suggested Reading

Leung RS, Biswas SV, Duncan M et al. (2008) Imaging features of von Hippel-Lindau disease. Radiographics. 28 (1): 65–79

Taouli B, Ghouadni M, Corréas JM et al. (2003) Spectrum of abdominal imaging findings in von Hippel-Lindau disease. AJR Am J Roentgenol.181 (4): 1049–54.

W

No Lemma

G. Zamboni, S. Gourtsoyianni, *MDCT and MRI of the Liver, Bile Ducts and Pancreas*, A-Z Notes in Radiological Practice and Reporting, DOI 10.1007/978-88-470-5720-3_23,

X

No Lemma

G. Zamboni, S. Gourtsoyianni, *MDCT and MRI of the Liver, Bile Ducts and Pancreas*, A-Z Notes in Radiological Practice and Reporting, DOI 10.1007/978-88-470-5720-3_24,

Y

No Lemma

G. Zamboni, S. Gourtsoyianni, *MDCT and MRI of the Liver, Bile Ducts and Pancreas*, A-Z Notes in Radiological Practice and Reporting, DOI 10.1007/978-88-470-5720-3_25,

Z

No Lemma

G. Zamboni, S. Gourtsoyianni, *MDCT and MRI of the Liver, Bile Ducts and Pancreas*, A-Z Notes in Radiological Practice and Reporting, DOI 10.1007/978-88-470-5720-3_26,